# HEMISPHERICITY AS A KEY TO UNDERSTANDING INDIVIDUAL DIFFERENCES

# HEMISPHERICITY AS A KEY TO UNDERSTANDING INDIVIDUAL DIFFERENCES

*Edited by*

**ISADORE L. SONNIER, B.A., M.Ed., Ed.D.**
*Professor of Science Education
University of Southern Mississippi
Hattiesburg, Mississippi*

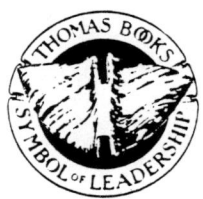

**CHARLES C THOMAS • PUBLISHER**
*Springfield • Illinois • U.S.A.*

*Published and Distributed Throughout the World by*
CHARLES C THOMAS • PUBLISHER
2600 South First Street
Springfield, Illinois 62794-9265

This book is protected by copyright. No part of
it may be reproduced in any manner without
written permission from the publisher.

© *1992 by* CHARLES C THOMAS • PUBLISHER
ISBN 0-398-05766-4
Library of Congress Catalog Card Number: 91-32019

*With* THOMAS BOOKS *careful attention is given to all details of manufacturing and design. It is the Publisher's desire to present books that are satisfactory as to their physical qualities and artistic possibilities and appropriate for their particular use.* THOMAS BOOKS *will be true to those laws of quality that assure a good name and good will.*

*Printed in the United States of America*
*SC-R-3*

**Library of Congress Cataloging-in-Publication Data**

Hemisphericity as a key to understanding individual differences / edited by Isadore L. Sonnier.
    p. cm.
  Includes bibliographical references and index.
  ISBN 0-398-05766-4 (hard)
  1. Personality—Physiological aspects. 2. Cerebral dominance.
3. Individual differences. 4. Personality and occupation.
I. Sonnier, Isadore L.
BF698.9.B5H46  1992
155.2'2—dc20
                                                91-32019
                                                    CIP

# CONTRIBUTORS

**MARY ANN ADAMS, B.A., M.S., Ph.D.**
*Assistant Professor of Family Relations*
*University of Southern Mississippi*
*Hattiesburg, Mississippi*

**JAMES J. ASHER, B.A., M.A., Ph.D.**
*Professor of Psychology*
*San Jose State University*
*San Jose, California*

**WALTER W. FREY, B.E.E.**
*Research Engineer*
*The Accelerator Department*
*Brookhaven National Laboratory*
*Upton, New York*

**JEAN A. HASPESLAGH, B.S.N., M.S.Ed., M.S., D.N.S.**
*Associate Professor of Nursing*
*University of Southern Mississippi*
*Hattiesburg, Mississippi*

**G. RICHARD LARKIN, B.A., M.U.R.Pl.**
*Assistant Professor of Geography and Area Development*
*Director of Community and Regional Planning*
*University of Southern Mississippi*
*Hattiesburg, Mississippi*

**MARTHA J. LARKIN, B.S., M.S., M.Ed.**
*Special Education Teacher*
*Rawls Spring Elementary School*
*Hattiesburg, Mississippi*

**MARK McELROY, B.A. M.A., Assistant Editor**
*Visiting Instructor of English*
*University of Southern Mississippi*
*Hattiesburg, Mississippi*

**THOMAS R. PANKO, B.A., M.A., Ph.D.**
*Associate Professor of Criminal Justice*
*University of Southern Mississippi*
*Hattiesburg, Mississippi*

**W. HARVEY POOLE, III, B.S., M.S.**
*Assistant to the Director,*
*School of Human Performance and Recreation*
*Instructor of Physical Education*
*University of Southern Mississippi*
*Hattiesburg, Mississippi*

**WILLIAM C. SMITH, B.S., M.B.A., D.B.A.**
*Assistant Professor of Marketing*
*University of Southern Mississippi*
*Hattiesburg, Mississippi*

**CLAUDINE B. SONNIER, B.S., M.S., Ed.S.**
*Home Economics Teacher*
*Forrest County Agricultural High School*
*Brooklyn, Mississippi*

**DAVID. L. SONNIER, B.S.**
*Graduate Student in Computing Science*
*Georgia Institute of Technology*
*Atlanta, Georgia*

**ISADORE L. SONNIER, B.A., M.Ed., Ed.D., EDITOR**
*Professor of Science Education*
*University of Southern Mississippi*
*Hattiesburg, Mississippi*

**JOHN S. SONNIER, B.S.**
*Sales Representative*
*Ortho Pharmaceutical Corporation*
*Baritan, New Jersey*

**ARTHUR R. SOUTHERLAND, B.M.Ed., M.Ed., Ph.D.**
*Professor of Educational Leadership and Research*
*University of Southern Mississippi*
*Hattiesburg, Mississippi*

**JAMES H. C. THOMAS, Jr., B.S., J.D.**
*Attorney at Law*
*Hattiesburg, Mississippi*

**ANDREA L. WESLEY, B.A., M.A., Ph.D.**
*Associate Professor of Psychology*
*University of Southern Mississippi*
*Hattiesburg, Mississippi*

**JOSEPH W. WESLEY, B.S., M.Ed.**
*Graduate Student in Counselor Education*
*College of Education*
*Mississippi State University*
*Mississippi State, Mississippi*

**EDDY L. WHEELER, B.S., M.S.**
*Assistant Professor of Journalism*
*University of Southern Mississippi*
*Hattiesburg, Mississippi*

**HAMPTON S. WILLIAMS, B.S., Ed.M., Ed.D.**
*Associate Professor of Educational Leadership and Research*
*University of Southern Mississippi*
*Hattiesburg, Mississippi*

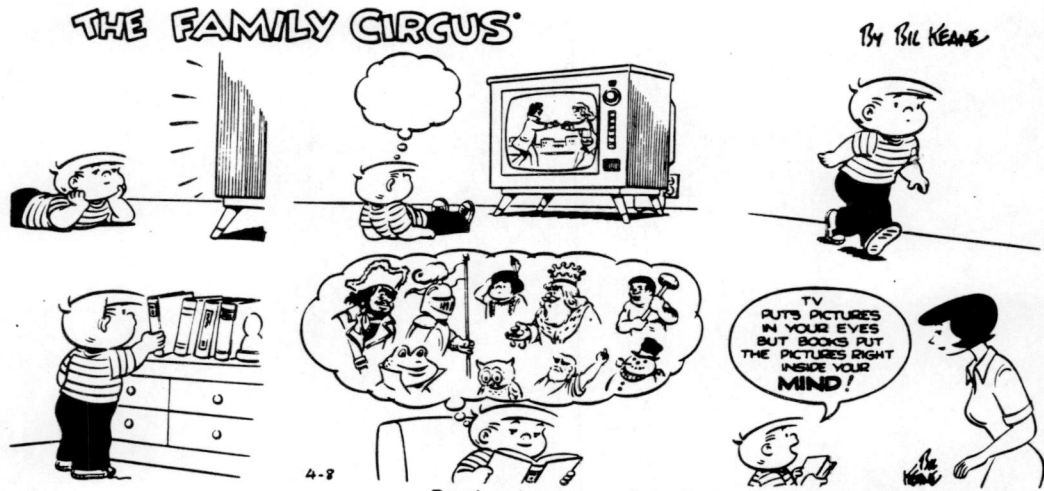

# PREFACE

The cerebral hemisphericity phenomenon, through its overtly expressed hemispheric preference (HP) activities, is suggested to be a major contributor to individual differences in personality development among humans. Properly understood and implemented, this knowledge has the potential to remediate strife and disruptive confrontations in all of the institutions of human interaction. For example, in educational thought and practice, knowledge and understanding of the universal role of HP has the potential for revealing not only *how* to reach and teach more students—but can also help us realize *why* we must do so. However, its implementation is plagued with misconceptions.

A cursory examination of the spectrum of HP expressions reveals two sets of antagonistic value systems. Both are needed in order to liberate reality so as to come to grips with common cause, negotiated to common good. Dialogue, ranging from casual conversation to constructive confrontation, is an absolute necessity in due course of proper institutional management. Allowed, or even tolerated, dialogue brings unity in educational, political, social, economic, and all other human institutions.

However, if dialogue is disallowed, avoided, suppressed, or rejected as due process in institutional management, an atmosphere of disunity, dishonesty, and corruption is created, eventually leading to disruptive and even destructive confrontation. No institution or society can survive without the democratizing touch of both liberal and conservative input. History clearly teaches that institutional management with only conservative HP input sets into motion monologue over dialogue, generating only policies and services that are neither with common cause nor for common good. For a quick analysis or handy reminder of this, consider the trend in politics and education, in which the policy-and-practice pendulum swings from one bungling, antagonistic side to the other.

The HP phenomenon is suggested to be the major influence on institutional management. Given the tenet that education is the main artery of sustenance for all other human institutions, *holistic education* is a test of its applicability. When both visual and analytical thought processing propensities of the hemispheric phenomenon are stimulated simultaneously and concurrently, it is tantamount to reaching and teaching both hemispheres, the whole mind, or the whole person.

This teaching strategy has been shown to have the potential to compensate for HP differences in both teaching and learning styles. While nurturing analytical thought processing and skill development in visual learners, holistic education nurtures visual thought processing and skill development in analytical learners as well. By infusing meaning and responsibility into the educational process, holistic education approaches the ultimate goal of education—to educate all students—more completely than traditional models.

Because of its all-encompassing role over other institutions, education is probably the best place to start the healing process by implementing the knowledge, understanding, and power of dialogue. It is sorely needed everywhere as a possible cure for disruptive and destructive confrontations, often an elitist-egalitarian struggle, that weaken all of our democratic institutions.

Conservatives argue for status quo. However, the role of confrontation has never before been known or understood as not only a tool, but a necessity for different input by different values as a check and balance system. Dialogue in constructive confrontation is the essence of civilization and the crux of a democracy. The history of man's search for socialization is littered with the monologue of conservative, authoritarian gluttony for political power and economic greed.

The project that produced this book had as its main goal the exploration of not only the volatile issues, but the degree of unity or disunity precipitated by the antagonistic nature of HP values. Attention was paid to the contributions of HP toward more effective ways of institutional management. Given success in describing the *nature and role of HP* in individual differences, exploring the more elusive *nurturing* of these different individuals in personality development and self-esteem was also a goal.

I.L.S.

# INTRODUCTION

My entire career as an educator has been spent wrestling with and struggling toward a better understanding of individual differences among my students. With the advent and knowledge of hemispheric preference came this better understanding of not only visual and analytical students, but also of how the same perceptual differences divide teachers and bring disunity, disruption, and even failure to this important institution.

I repeat these comments made in the introduction of my last book, published by Charles C Thomas, *Methods and Techniques of Holistic Education.* This is the story of my continuing struggle to communicate the fact that students have hemispheric preference differences. Further, they have the right and the need to freely develop in these naked and basic differences. A model has emerged which I think has the potential to revolutionize education. However, the very thought of a revolution is threatening to a conservative leadership. Further, the hemispheric phenomenon is in itself a continuing source of disagreement because of the different vantage points due to these different hemispheric preferences. However, these differences most often emerge as differences due to semantics. Having a visual preference causes one to see the world differently than do those with an analytical preference.

Thus, those in leadership positions in any social institution are encouraged to sift through the ideas and suggestions of this book. Each is encouraged to draw personal conclusions concerning how to become a more effective leader by applying the knowledge of hemisphericity from a personal vantage point. Different leaders will draw different conclusions, a fact that adds credibility to these considerations.

I am grateful for the assistance of the many contributors toward the establishment of hemisphericity as a vital force in institutional management. Together we wish for each and every leader to try these ideas out for themselves. In that education has an all-encompassing role as the basis for all of the other institutions, educators are invited to investigate the utility of holistic education in the microteaching environment. Clearly, we can all improve when it comes to teaching and reaching a greater population of students. Reaching ALL students approaches the impossible — but not trying to reach them is unthinkable.

I.L.S.

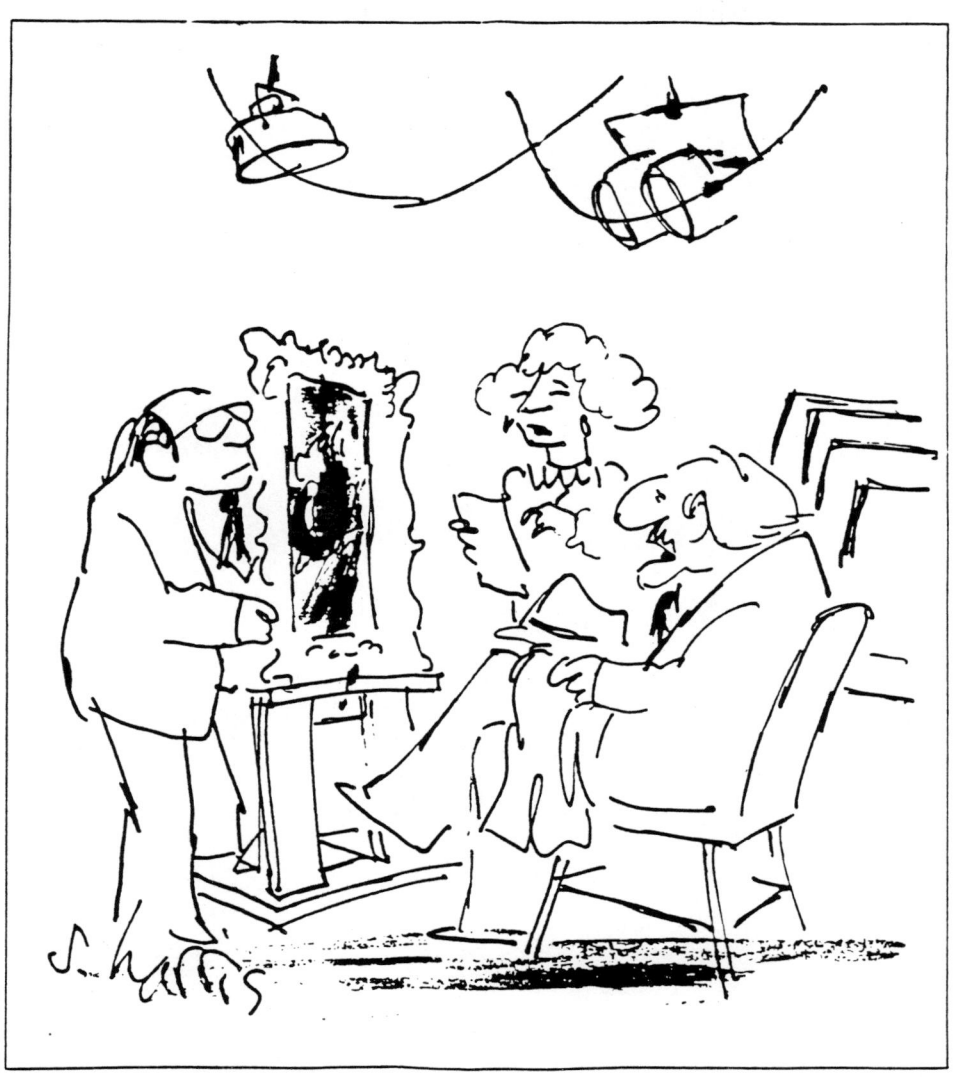

"On some, my right brain says they're good art, but my left brain says they're bad investments. On others, my right brain says they're bad art, but my left brain says they're good investments."
Published by Sigma XI, The Scientific Research Society. Courtesy Sidney Harris.

# ACKNOWLEDGMENTS

Many have contributed to the success of this project and to this book on how individual differences contribute to institutional management. I am most grateful to Mark McElroy, our assistant editor, for his remarkable ability to wear the two hats of truth. He is blessed with not only the sense of vision and overseeing, but with the skill for penetrating analysis of the minutest details as well.

I also express appreciation to all of the contributors who took time out from their busy schedules to witness hemispheric preference in themselves and in their various professions. We all wish for this project to bring a better understanding of that human nature which is basic to hemispheric preference and how it can be better understood in all of the institutions that serve us. But, we acknowledge that the project is not finished. It needs to continue to grow and to be developed by others who also have the need and vision to nurture this better understanding of how hemispheric preference contributes to individual differences and to institutional management.

I.L.S.

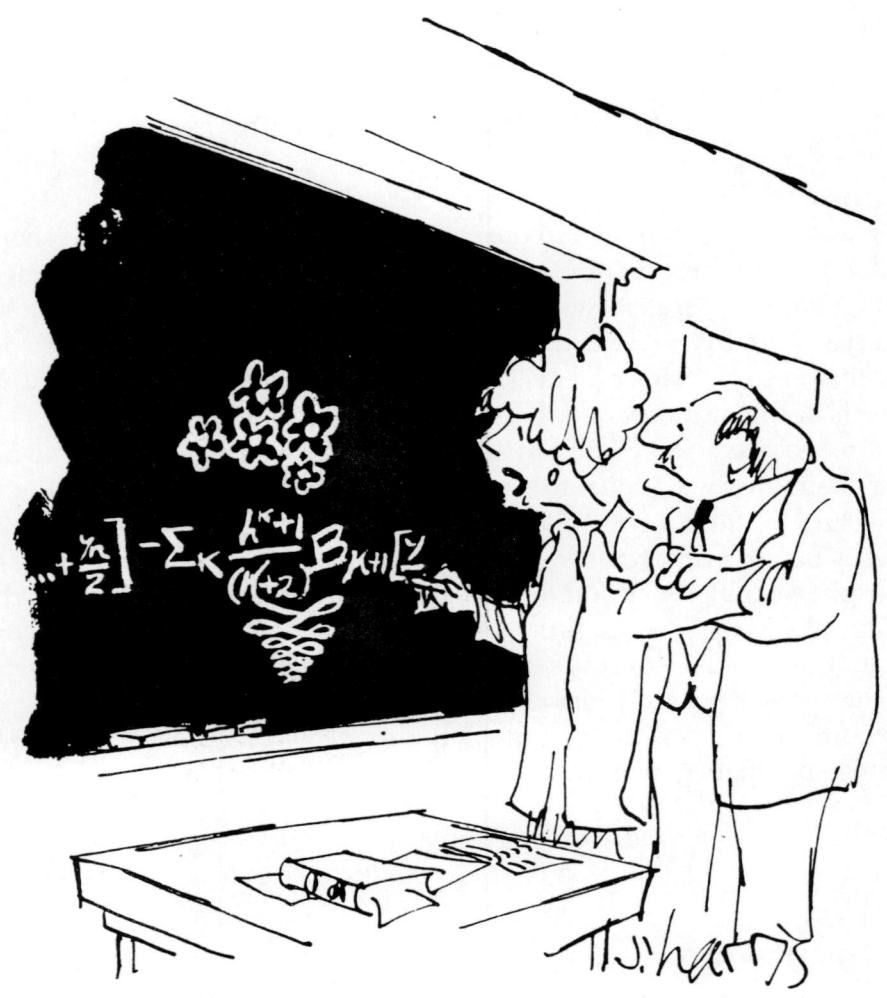

"Every once in a while my right brain throws something in."

**Published by Sigma XI, The Scientific Research Society. Courtesy Sidney Harris.**

# CONTENTS

|  | Page |
|---|---|
| *Preface* | ix |
| *Introduction* | xi |

*Chapter*

1. The Two Sides of Truth
   *Isadore L. Sonnier* ............................................. 3
2. Hemisphericity as a Key to
   Understanding Individual Differences
   *Isadore L. Sonnier* ............................................. 6
3. The Sonnier Model of Hemispheric Preference
   *Isadore L. Sonnier* ............................................. 9
4. Investigating the Hemispheric Preferences
   of the Social Styles
   *Isadore L. Sonnier and Andrea L. Wesley* ..................... 14
5. Visual and Analytical Thought Processing
   *Isadore L. Sonnier and Mark McElroy* ......................... 18
6. Conservatism vs. the "L–Word":
   An Explanation of HP in Human Institutions
   *Isadore L. Sonnier and James J. Asher* ....................... 25
7. The Sonnier Model of Educational Management:
   Implementing Holistic Education
   *Isadore L. Sonnier and Claudine B. Sonnier* .................. 30
8. Hemispheric Preference in Education
   *Isadore L. Sonnier* ........................................... 36
9. Instructional Supervision for Holistic Education
   *Hampton S. Williams* .......................................... 39
10. Relationship between Hemispheric Preference
    and Standardized Testing
    *Arthur R. Southerland* ....................................... 48
11. A Brain Drain in the Engineering Sciences
    *Walter W. Frey* .............................................. 52

12. Hemispheric Preference Among Scientists
    *Isadore L. Sonnier* .............................. 56
13. Hemispheric Preference as a Factor
    in Public Policy Formulation
    *G. Richard Larkin* .............................. 59
14. Hemispheric Preference in the Rise and Fall of a Business
    *William C. Smith* ............................... 63
15. Hemispheric Preference in Moral Theology
    *Isadore L. Sonnier* .............................. 67
16. Hemispheric Preference and Crime
    *Thomas R. Panko* ............................... 72
17. Hemispheric Preference Among Athletic Administrators
    *W. Harvey Poole, III* ............................ 75
18. Hemispheric Preference in Military Leadership
    *David L. Sonnier* ............................... 78
19. Hemispheric Preference in Photojournalism Education
    *Eddy L. Wheeler* ................................ 82
20. Hemispheric Preference Awareness in Public Education
    *Martha J. Larkin* ............................... 85
21. Hemispheric Preference as a Factor in
    Stress Management Among Nurses
    *Jean A. Haspeslagh* .............................. 91
22. The Role of Hemispheric Preference in Law Practice
    *James H. C. Thomas, Jr.* ......................... 95
23. The Social Aspects of Hemisphericity in Education
    *Andrea L. Wesley* ............................... 99
24. The Role of Hemispheric Preference in
    Sales Representative Training
    *John S. Sonnier* ................................ 102
25. The Role of Hemispheric Preference in
    Understanding Family Systemic Functioning
    *Mary Ann Adams* ............................... 108
26. An Historical Perspective of Hemispheric Preference
    in Counseling
    *Joseph W. Wesley and Isadore L. Sonnier* ........ 113

*Bibliography* ......................................... 119
*Index* ............................................... 123

# LIST OF FIGURES

*Figure*                                                                             *Page*

1. The Hemispheric Preference of Selected Life-Styles ........ 10
2. The Universal Views Resulting from Visual and Analytical Thought Processing ............................. 13
3. Investigating the Hemispheric Preferences of the Social Styles ........................................... 15
4. The Hemispheric Preference of Selected Life-Styles ........ 20
5. How the Analytical Hemisphere Processes Information ...... 26
6. How the Visual Hemisphere Process Information .......... 26
7. How to Communicate with Each Hemisphere .............. 27
8. Four Categories of Cognitive Achievement/Affective Attainment ............................................ 31
9. Student Checklist for Cognitive Achievement/Affective Attainment ............................................ 32
10. Four Categories of Students' Evaluation of Teaching ........ 33
11. Form for Collecting Data on Cognitive Achievement/Affective Attainment Traditional Teaching vs. Holistic Teaching ............... 34
12. Form for the Maintenance of Cognitive Achievement/Affective Attainment in *Category 1* ........... 35
13. The Four Categories of Teacher-Success in the Sonnier Model of Educational Management ........... 41
14. The Universal Views Resulting from Visual and Analytical Thought Processing ................ 70
15. The Universal Views Resulting from Visual and Analytical Thought Processing ................ 110

# HEMISPHERICITY AS A KEY TO UNDERSTANDING INDIVIDUAL DIFFERENCES

# Chapter 1

# THE TWO SIDES OF TRUTH

Isadore L. Sonnier

There once lived a great people who would gather every year from every corner of the land to celebrate The Bruhaha, an event of infinite and incredible importance.

Some collected sand and pebbles and dragged massive stones great distances so as to form and erect monuments to commemorate these events of infinite and incredible importance.

"Why do you bother?" said others. "Why strain yourselves with such burdens as to leave so many of you haggard, tired and ill? Today's problems are much more in need of your care."

For their conservative ways, the monument builders became known as Cons, and the cynical, liberal critics were called Libs. As the years passed, the two groups differed more and more in their views and feelings about things.

The Cons' festivals grew and grew. How proud they were to celebrate, make speeches and commemorate The Bruhaha. This was the event of greatest importance and was remembered here and there, throughout the land, by those who *knew the man* who *knew the man* who did this, that, or the other.

The Libs were thought to be confused, ill informed, and ignorant because they questioned far and wide, asking to learn *exactly*, "What is The Bruhaha? When or where did it take place?" They questioned exactly who did what, only to be told of the man who *knew of the man* who did this, that, or the other.

"Where is your patriotism?" said the Cons to the Libs. "Why can't you behave with respect and love for men who did so much for your land?"

Said the Libs to the Cons, "We are too busy taking care of your sick, lame and lazy to be bothered with the history of such a mystery."

| "If you are so concerned about the sick, why do you support the killing of the unborn?" asked the Cons. | "Our belief and support of individual rights should neither be a reflection of our ethics nor of our theology," responded the Libs. |

The squabbles grew from name calling and shouting, over the years, until one day a full blown riot erupted. The people were angered to the point of siding, brothers against brothers and families against families. A civil war left people hurt and drained and the land in ruin.

| Libs were captured and made to learn the rules, etiquette, and the ethics of the Cons. | Cons were captured and not made to learn the rules, etiquette, and the ethics of the Libs. |

When these people were down and demoralized, there appeared two leaders, one who offered them the power, strength, and peace of mind of a centralized government. The other offered them a voice in their government with individual, self-determination and collective bargaining. At this time, the latter captured a collective imagination and commanded the attention of all.

Said he, "We fight, to stand tall in dignity and personal pride. We battle each other with little concern that it is each other we bruise and hurt. Thus, we have destroyed our land, squandered our wealth, and are all in poor physical and mental health.

"Instead, I suggest we use our energies to build together. We should use our similarities to gain strength and with our differences, develop wisdom. For, from our similarities we will build fibers of unity and from our differences we will build the fabric of our liberty." The words of this man were heard.

| The Cons took stock of the here and now and started construction so as to build houses and grow crops for wealth. And, with personal prosperity, they built hospitals and banks in which to store this great wealth. | The Libs pitched in to build schools to free minds from ignorance, to build houses for comfort and shelter, grow crops for food, and to build hospitals for good health. They built banks, all of these as monuments to great wealth and prosperity. |

In time, they grew to be a great people who would gather every year from every corner of the land to celebrate The Bruhaha, an event of infinite and incredible importance.

Some collected sand and pebbles and dragged massive stones great distances so as to form and erect monuments to commemorate these events of infinite and incredible importance.

"Why do you bother?" said others. "Why strain yourselves with such burdens as to leave so many of you haggard, tired and ill? Today's problems are much more in need of your care."

## Chapter 2

# HEMISPHERICITY AS A KEY TO UNDERSTANDING INDIVIDUAL DIFFERENCES

ISADORE L. SONNIER

In its brief history, the study and knowledge of human cerebral hemisphericity has not only attracted much attention among educators, but has created a notable amount of controversy (Gardner, 1978; Gazzaniga, 1975; Keefe, 1982; Nebes, 1975; Sonnier, 1982a, 1982b, 1984, 1985, 1989). Even so, many researchers are seeking ways to find more of these hemispheric specializations and to establish ways in which to apply this knowledge to their own academic activities. *Hemisphericity*, or the hemispheric preference (HP) phenomenon, may be one of the most important factors to consider when seeking a better understanding of our own individual differences. These are the same differences reflected in our collective differences and manifested, through social and political interactions, in all of our institutions. A review of selected literature is discussed concerning the status of the research and development of HP (see Chap. 3 for more discussion and personal observations).

**Discovery of The Hemisphericity.** Hemisphericity is the term implying "the intriguing possibility that individuals have a tendency to appeal to one hemisphere and its mode of thought more than the other . . . a term borrowed from Bogen (et al., 1972)," according to Krashen (1977, p. 121). However, significant misunderstandings have obstructed the utility and applicability of the hemisphericity phenomenon in education. The first was quick to surface. Because of the high level of sympathetic consciousness with analytical processing, the left hemisphere was immediately dubbed the *major hemisphere*. However, due either to the subliminal nature or the lack of importance of visual and nonverbal processing, or both, the right hemisphere was relegated to be the *subordinate, minor hemisphere*. While there is yet a hint of this lingering confusion, the propensities of both hemispheres are today widely accepted as equally important and orchestrated entities that contribute to thought processing.

The second obstacle is the perpetuated misconception by an educational system which not only ignores the utility of visual functions and processes, but debates the validity of hemisphericity on the basis of flawed data (Sonnier, 1982a, 1984, 1989). From the onset of these discoveries, in Nebes' (1975) words, "perhaps we are short-changing ourselves when we educate only left-sided talents in basic schooling... the inverse relationship between scholastic achievement and creativity... overtraining for verbal skills at the expense of nonverbal abilities" (p. 16).

**The HP Phenomenon.** The natural division of the brain into the right and left hemispheres has long been a cause for speculation among researchers in behavior and learning. The *split-brain* research, as it has come to be called, was initiated in 1960 when Dr. Joseph Bogen proposed that the brain be split (the corpus callosum sectioned) "for the purpose of controlling the interhemispheric spread of epilepsy" (Gazzaniga, 1975, p. 10). From observing these patients, Bogen (1977) recognized a dichotomy which "has a sound physiologic basis... (with) two principal and different types of cognition, each typically identifiable with one of the two cerebral hemispheres" (p. 137). Each is the seat of complex sets of operations, orchestrating the thought processes and body functions.

Further observation of these patients revealed a dichotomy, described by Nebes (1975) as, "symbolic versus visual-spatial, associative versus apperceptive, propositional versus appositional, and analytic versus gestalt (suggesting)... that the organization and processing of data by the right hemisphere is in predisposition for perceiving the total rather than the parts. By contrast, the left hemisphere is seen to analyze input sequentially, abstracting out the relevant details and associating these with verbal symbols" (p. 15).

Witelson (1977) explained the common knowledge that nonreaders are predominantly visually-oriented persons. She found evidence that children with developmental dyslexia possessed two visual hemispheres rather than one of each. This possibility lends unexpected credence to the probability that highly analytical individuals have two analytical hemispheres rather than one of each. Evidence reveals this parameter to be a normal curve distribution with small populations of visual and analytical persons at both ends and the eclectic orchestration of these two extremes in the rest of the population (Sonnier, 1982a, 1982b, 1984, 1985, 1989).

**Factors That Obstruct Research, Development and Application of HP.** In reviewing Vitale (1982) and Williams (1983), it became apparent that throughout the literature, it is widely accepted that visual persons learn *visually* and that analytical persons learn *auditorily*. The assumption is that those who make better grades are better listeners. This refers to the senses, visual and auditory, and is therefore misleading. Reference should be made to the hemispheric preference modes, *visual and analytical.* Personal observation and experience suggests that, when motivated, visual students are not only acutely auditory, but become voracious learners.

This may explain why it is difficult to use student achievement as a determination for hemispheric preference. These data are most often rather bland in that not all analytical persons are good students, nor are all visual persons poor students. For example, in noting the results portrayed in the 1989 popular movie, *Stand and Deliver,* the high level of achievement by all of the students made it difficult to distinguish between visual and analytical students. For these reasons, reference should be made to the hemispheric processes—whether one is a visual or an analytical learner—rather than to the sensory processes—visual and auditory—as to the loci of learning experiences or the seat of learning styles, as well as social styles, teaching modes, or, in all probability, most other traits should be made to the HP phenomenon.

## Conclusion

Aside from any discussion of *nurture,* or environmental factors, that contribute to personality development and individual differences, hemisphericity is in all probability the *nature* key to understanding the apparent dichotomy of individual differences among human beings. An outstanding implication for the HP phenomenon is that *truth has two sets of values, the visual approach and the analytical approach, and that both are needed to liberate its reality.* Unfortunately, the literature appears to be flawed with misconceptions that prevent progress in either the implementation or application of this phenomenon.

# Chapter 3

# THE SONNIER MODEL OF HEMISPHERIC PREFERENCE

Isadore L. Sonnier

The Sonnier Model of Hemispheric Preference (SMHP) was formulated from data and evidence that hemispheric preference (HP) is the basis for the common thread of individual differences among human beings (Sonnier, 1982b, 1985, 1989). This determination is obtained from self-diagnosis of individuals who are very sure that they are visual and not at all analytical, referred to as highly visual (7%), those who are very sure that they are analytical and not at all visual (highly analytical, 7%), those who do both but are more visual than analytical (slightly visual, 40%), those who do both but are more analytical than visual (slightly analytical, 40%), and those who do not know their hemispheric preference and cannot respond to these questions (presumed nondominant, 6%) (see Fig. 1).

Deviation from these results may come from a nonrandom sample or from an inexperienced sample. An example of a nonrandom sample is a group of elementary school teachers. Evidence is that approximately 70 percent of all inservice and preservice elementary school teachers are visually-oriented. It is also my experience that most groups sampled can be categorized as inexperienced because of the large number of people who have never before made this determination. However, given this information and the same questions two or three weeks later improves towards a normal distribution of these data.

Further, it is my observation that if the hemispheric preference phenomenon has to be explained to someone, no amount of explanation will suffice. The only scientific evidence that can be offered is that a small population of people are self-diagnosed visual and not at all analytical and another small population of people are self-diagnosed analytical and not at all visual. While most others claim to do both, but admit doing one more than the other, those in need of an explanation appear to be void of this awareness.

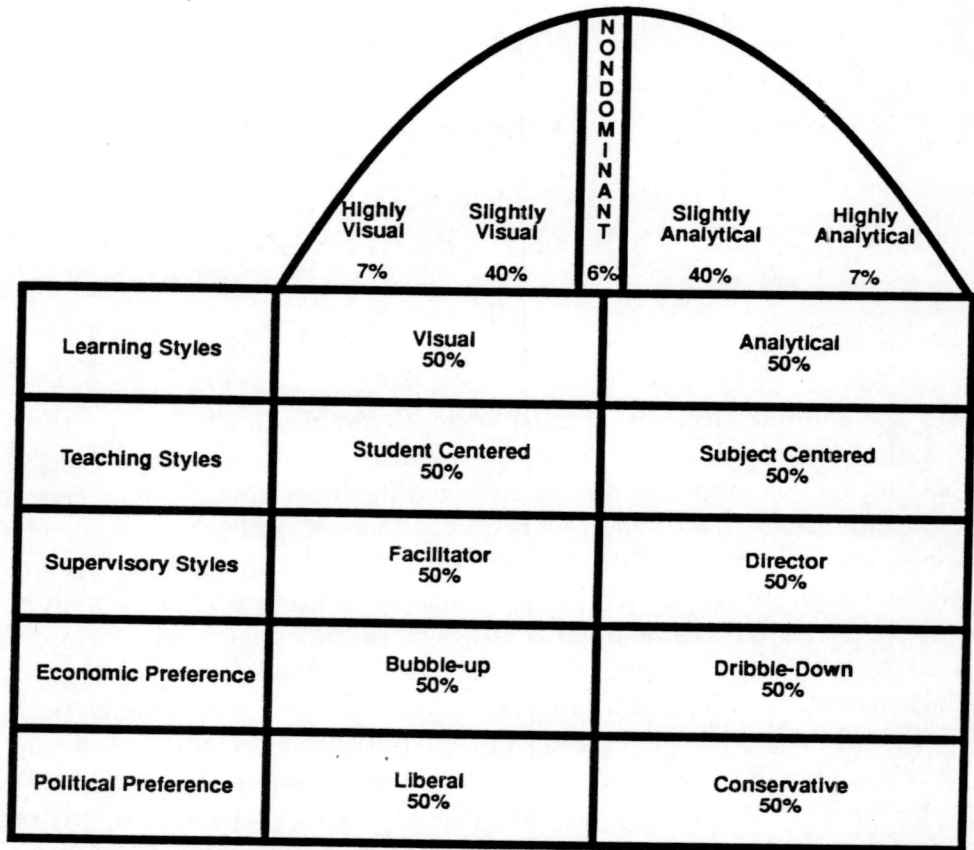

**THE HEMISPHERIC PREFERENCES OF SELECTED LIFE-STYLES**

*Figure 1.* These are but a few of the life styles that are directly influenced by HP and will have to be better understood before coming to grips with such intervening variables as "low-esteem" and other detractors to positive self-actualization. However, evidence is that either because of nature, nurture, or both, visual persons are more commonly prone to low self-esteem syndrome than are analytical persons (Adapted from Sonnier, I.L., 1982b, 1985, 1989).

There is yet another factor that may occasionally prevent the obtaining of normally distributed data from this self-diagnosis technique. Visual thought processing appears to be more consciously pronounced than analytical processing. This factor may contribute to an excessive skewing of these data toward the visual side.

**Misnomer Obstructing HP Knowledge.** There is a factor that has obstructed research and development of the HP knowledge. A review of this literature reveals that it is widely and mistakenly accepted that visual persons are called *visual learners* and that analytical persons are called *auditory learners*. Reference is made to the senses, eyes and ears, rather than to the two HPs, *visual* and *analytical*. Data on "visual and auditory" were inconclusive because the wrong question was posed and the baby was thrown out with the bathwater.

**HP Among Teachers.** Sonnier (1975, 1976) described these differences as "constructive and creative." Today, he believes the constructive process to be the analytical hemisphere's way of exploring and pioneering new frontiers. Much as an engineer is well suited for building bridges and structures to meet any given need, this thinking is limited to the linear logical processing of that person's wealth of background knowledge. Coming up with "new structures" is a delimitation in this processing system. However, creativity is well established as being linked with visualization, the forte of the visual hemisphere. As with the SMHP structures herein described, the "constructivity and creativity" data were obtained from self-diagnosis of elementary and secondary school teachers.

**HP Among Learners.** In a rural or farm environment, highly visual children grow up probing nature by kicking over rotting logs and stumps, observing animal behavior and growing plants. By so doing, they develop an understanding of nature and of the real world. Evidence is that these children do poorly, for example, in a biology course when emphasis is placed on verbalizing in abstractions. However, given the scenario of not only growing up probing nature, but having a set of picture books with which to relate these experiences into the abstractions of language, the same children could become academically adept.

Meanwhile, analytical children grow up reading everything that they can put their hands on, including encyclopedias. They, too, know more than some of their teachers, on occasion. And, as with highly visual children, they could become either obstinate, disruptive, or reclusive, and could also do poorly in school. The disturbing reality is that the visual tots that live in urban areas and have no old logs or rotten stumps to kick over and many analytical tots have no books to read. It is socially improper for rural girls to go around kicking over stumps. The bottom line is that the nature-nurture relationship of the HP phenomenon is complex and deeply in need of further clarification so as to identify areas in need of investigation.

**The HP Phenomenon in General.** Although the HP differences of the

SMHP can be clearly laid out as differences that are generated from two, mutually exclusive sources, visual and analytical thought processing, only the few highly visual and highly analytical individuals will consistently and exclusively reflect the decision making characteristics of their respective sources. The most likely situation is to find orchestrated adaptations of these extremes in different degrees and in various ways.

An interesting development concerning the SMHP that can be reported is the fact that when contributors were solicited for this book, only one out of about 12 scholars approached could actually say, "I know exactly what you want," and came up with a contribution. Most of the contributors appear to be visual. One impression was that analytical persons found discussion of the HP phenomenon to be uncomplementary or offensive. However, the most common impression was that the large population of mixed dominance people did not sufficiently understand HP to participate.

A dichotomy of these extremes, adapted from Gula (1989), reveals the characteristics, methods of operation, advantages, and disadvantages of HP. Although one system is not considered better or worse than, or superior or inferior to the other, each has definite advantages and disadvantages. Some of these traits are gifts of nature's strengths. Others may be weaknesses in need of nurturing towards positive and improved personality development (see Fig. 2).

Given the present understanding of HP, the assumption is that people are evenly divided as analyticals and visuals. Visual teachers are student-oriented, and as supervisors of instruction, they are facilitators. In politics they are the liberals who advocate the bubble-up way of tax dispensation. Analytical teachers are subject-centered and, as supervisors of instruction, they are more direct in leadership. They are the conservatives in politics and prefer to see tax money dispensed among those who already possess economic power. Among many other subtle areas of HP differences are arts and crafts and science and technology. The differences become more obvious when visual and analytical people discuss such topics as arts vs. crafts, science vs. technology, liberal vs. conservatism, democratic vs. authoritarian leadership, or egalitarian vs. elitist rule.

Although further research will be needed to understand the role of HP as the influence of *nature* on personality development, even more elusive is the role of HP on *nurturing* and personality development.

| FEATURES | ANALYTICAL | VISUAL |
|---|---|---|
| CHARACTERISTICS | Views the world as complete and fixed for eternity. | Views a dynamic and evolving world through historical development. |
| | The world is marked by harmony of an objective order. | The world is marked by progressive growth and change. |
| | Speaks of the world in terms of well-defined essences using abstract, universal terms. | Speaks of the world in terms of individual traits using concrete historical concepts. |
| METHOD OF OPERATION | Begins with the abstract and derives principles from universal essence. | Begins with experience and derives accumulated experience. |
| | Deals with universals of humanhood by deriving principles from the physical nature of being human. | Deals eith the historical person in historically particular circumstances |
| | Conforms to authority and to pre-established norms. | Formulations of norms are historically conditioned |
| | Emphasis on duty and obligation to reproduce established order. | Emphasis on responsibility and actions fitting to changing times. |
| | Primarily deductive. | Primary inductive. |
| | Conclusions will remain the same. | Some conclusions will change as emperical evidence changes |
| | Conclusions are always secure as long as deductive logic is correct. | Leaving room for incompleteness, possible error, open to revision; conclusions are as accurate as evidence will allow, but these are accurate enough. |
| ADVANTAGES | Clear, simple, and sure on views of reality an conclusions about what to do. | Respects the uniquesness of the person and the peculiarities of historical circumstances |
| DISADVANTAGES | Tends to be authoritarian in the sense of claimimg to have answers suitable for all times. | Tends to be relative in the sense that everything is conditioned. |
| | Tends to be dogmatic in the sense of having the last word. | Tends to be antinomian in the sense that all laws are relative. |

## THE UNIVERSAL VIEWS RESULTING FROM VISUAL AND ANALYICAL THOUGHT PROCESSING

*Figure 2.* Visual and analytical HPs can be clearly delineated as the basis for the chemistry of group dynamics. The two different hemispheres generate mutually exclusive, universal views that in turn reflect their respective sources in document production. For example, analytical people tend to formulate conservative documents while visual people tend to formulate liberally-oriented documents. However, given the benefit of values input from both views, the product will in different degrees and in various ways be of greater benefit to all concerned (adapted from Gula, R.M., 1989, pp. 32–33).

## Chapter 4

# INVESTIGATING THE HEMISPHERIC PREFERENCES OF THE SOCIAL STYLES

ISADORE L. SONNIER AND ANDREA L. WESLEY

An exploratory instrument was developed to test the relationship between the Sonnier Model of Hemispheric Preference (SMHP) and the concept of social styles (SS). The previous investigation of this relationship utilized the Social Styles Profile of the Wilson Learning Corporation as the model for defining the concept of social styles (Lashbrook & Lashbrook, 1980; Sonnier, 1989, Chap. 29). It was hoped that the global, intuitive nature of the exploratory instrument could lead to answers to the relationship between hemispheric preference (HP) and SS which could be more clearly defined at a later date. This pilot investigation was an "adventure" to seek ways both to pose future research questions and to find possible answers.

Three tests were designed as parts of an exploratory instrument to make these determinations (see Fig. 3). The respondent's HP was established in Part I by selecting one from the gamut of HPs, from highly visual to highly analytical. Two assumptions were made from past experience with these data. Evidence is that people who neither know nor understand these questions have both propensities, but in a nonalignment mode. In addition, to utilize both propensities with the same proficiency was also assumed to be a nondominant characteristic. These assumptions were investigated in Part I (Fig. 3).

The choices (Items 1–6) were assigned the following weights for scoring:

| | |
|---|---|
| 1 = highly visual | (Item 1, see Fig. 3) |
| 2 = slightly visual | (Item 5) |
| 0 = don't understand these questions | (Item 3) |
| 3 = do both of these | (Item 4) |
| 4 = slightly analytical | (Item 6) |
| 5 = highly analytical | (Item 2). |

Major _____

Sex _____  Age _____  Classification: Fr____ So____ Jr____ Sr____ Gr____

**PART I. Definitions:**

To be **analytical** is to line up your thoughts and to use logic and reason.

To be **visual** is to see images of thoughts in your own mind.

**Using these definitions, SELECT ONE ANSWER FROM THE FIRST 6 ITEMS:**

1. I know that I am highly visual and not at all analytical.  _____
2. I know that I am highly analytical and not at all visual.  _____
3. I do not know or understand these questions.  _____
4. I do both with about the same proficiency.  _____
5. I do both but I am more visual than analytical.  _____
6. I do both but I am more analytical than visual.  _____

**PART II. SELECT ONE OF THE ENDINGS (a or b) TO COMPLETE ITEMS 7 AND 8:**

7. In response to other people, _____ .

    a. I am pushy and assertive.  _____
    b. I am passive and responsive.  _____

8. In dealing with new events in my life, _____ .

    a. I am versatile and accept new events, places and things.  _____
    b. It is hard for me to deal with new events, places and things.  _____

**PART III. RANK *A* THROUGH *D* TO COMPLETE ITEM 9.**

Rank 1 through 4, 1 = **MOST** descriptive and 4 = **LEAST** descriptive of me. Use each number once and please number each ending.

9. I think that other people see me as:

    A. Supportive Specialist: dependable, respectful, personable, conforming, retiring, non-commital, undisciplined, emotional.  _____

    B. Control Specialist: determined, thorough, decisive, efficient, pushy, tough-minded, dominating, harsh.  _____

    C. Social Specialist: personable, stimulating, enthusiastic, dramatic, inspiring, opinionated, promotional, undisciplined, excitable.  _____

    D. Technical Specialist: industrious, persistent, serious, vigilant, orderly, uncommunicative, indecisive, stuffy, exacting, impersonal.  _____

**INVESTIGATING THE HEMISPHERIC PREFERENCES OF THE SOCIAL STYLES**

*Figure 3.* Acting on the assumption that hemispheric preference is the root of all human behaviors, an attempt was made to impose hemisperic preference modes onto the social styles. Although there are too many built-in problems with these efforts to report success at this time, the efforts are nontheless worthy of sharing with the call for assistance (after Sonnier, 1989, see Chap. 29).

Part II was designed to determine the respondent's level of assertiveness (Item 7) and responsiveness (Item 8). Assertiveness and responsiveness have been found to be two variables which contribute greatly to one's social style (Lashbrook & Lashbrook, 1980, Sonnier, 1989, Chap. 29), The following characteristics are given for the SS, according to Sonnier (1989, Chap. 29):

— ANALYTICALS are lowly assertive (7b = 5) and lowly responsive (8b = 5).
— AMIABLES are lowly assertive (7b = 5) and highly responsive (8a = 1).
— DRIVERS are highly assertive (7a = 1) and lowly responsive (8b = 5).
— EXPRESSIVES are highly assertive (7a = 1) and highly responsive (8a = 1).

It is relatively apparent that the following equivalent relationships can be made between the SSs and the HPs. Indeed, that is the point of the investigation with this question (listed in the order as they appear on the questionnaire, see Fig. 3):

| SS | HP RELATIONSHIPS AND SCORING WEIGHTS: |
|---|---|
| Amiable | = Slightly Analytical ( = 4) or Slightly Visual ( = 2) |
| Driver | = Slightly Visual ( = 2) or Slightly Analytical ( = 4) |
| Expressive | = Highly Visual ( = 1) |
| Analytical | = Analytical ( = 5). |

In making the equivalent relationships, there is little doubt that the SS of being analytical is most similar to the HP of being analytical. Likewise, the expressive SS is most similar to a visual HP. However, it is less obvious that amiable is most similar to being slightly analytical and that driver is most similar to being slightly visual. Part III was designed to determine which SS, amiable or driver, is most like being slightly visual or slightly analytical.

To make this determination, respondents were asked to rank the four SSs, $A$ = amiable, $B$ = driver, $C$ = expressive, and $D$ = analytical, from 1 = most like me to 4 = least like me (see Fig. 3). In Part III of the test, the slightly analytical weight was 4 and that of slightly visual was 2. An expected result of Part III had the assumptions that slightly visual and slightly analytical persons are by nature one of these, but are easily nurtured with traits of the other. However, highly visual and highly analytical persons are less prone to adopt or adapt opposite traits by way of nurturing.

**Results.** This phase of the pilot investigation was not as fruitful as anticipated because of several internal problems. However, while the results did not support our operational research questions, the data did not negate the questions. For example, nearly half of the respondents were classified as amiable. This finding is assumed to be a reflection of the terms used as descriptors for the four SS characteristics. Also supportive of this assumption is the fact that very few respondents saw themselves as being analytical by these standards. Some problems were expected. For example, Sonnier (see Chap. 3) has found that people are more aware of having a visual preference than of having an analytical preference. He has also found that an inexperienced sample needs time to reflect and discern their SS or HP choice. Over the course of several months, as many as ten percent could change their choice several times (see Chap. 3). The influence of a nurturing environment could be an important factor in these stable or consistent choices. Also, with the present instrument, it was not possible to determine if indeed persons from one SS can adopt traits from the opposite SS.

Because this pilot investigation was not initially planned as a phase of the project that produced this book, time did not permit further study. An invitation is extended for others to help with these investigations. For example, the next phase could be to "tone down" the possible negative implied meanings of some of the analytical descriptors so as to make each choice one which the respondent can be proud of as a self-descriptor.

## Conclusion

The conclusion is that we are headed in the right direction with the assumption that the SSs are another way to express the HP phenomenon. An instrument is needed with a mode of application that will compensate for some of the internal problems that plagued the exploratory one used in this phase of these investigations.

## Chapter 5

## VISUAL AND ANALYTICAL THOUGHT PROCESSING

ISADORE L. SONNIER AND MARK MCELROY

*"Unity and diversity are two sides of the same coin."*
C. S. Lewis

Visual and analytical thought processing are discussed by an extremely visual person and a near center, slightly analytical swinger. Although many highly analytical persons were asked to make this representative statement, all approached declined. However, part of the message of this chapter is that doing so was neither needed nor necessary.

The underlying theme of this chapter is, as with the rest of the book, "Truth has two values and both are needed to liberate its reality." Although each HP has both assets and shortcomings, one system is neither better than nor superior to the other.

### Understanding the Two Preferences

At the heart of conflicts between the people who have different hemispheric preferences is a basic misunderstanding of each other. Visual people are perceived as a threat by analytical people because they do not easily conform and challenge established norms. Analytical persons, on the other hand, readily conform to established norms. Resolving the resulting conflicts can only be accomplished through more effective communications. To understand that HP is basic to individual differences is to recognize that out of this diversity comes the potential for greater unity.

Extremely visual and analytical people are presumed to possess two hemispheres of the same kind because of the evidence that these propensities appear to be mutually exclusive traits. By nature, extremely visual persons are not at all analytical and extremely analytical persons appear devoid of visual traits. However, highly visual individuals can be found performing highly analytical activities, such as crossword puzzles and word jumbles. Sonnier, for example, was a crytographer in the military service. However, it is his observation that one is less likely to find highly analytical persons performing highly visual activities.

The study of HP reveals a relatively small number of entirely visual or entirely analytical persons. The majority of persons display both of these traits in different areas of their lives. The resulting melange of preference disrupts our overall perception of exactly what hemispheric preference brings about, and those persons with equally divided or "ambidextrous" HP may not even be able to grasp the concept of HP differentiation. Individual difference traits result from the contributions of these two modes of perception (see Fig. 4).

## Understanding the Visual Preference

**Creativity.** It is both widely stated and commonly accepted that the visual hemisphere is the seat of long-term memory. If this is the case, it may contribute to creativity as the visual person's greatest asset. This may substantiate the appearance that visual thinking is supplied with a most vast source of information, making it easy to fill in missing parts of any mental picture. Visual people come up with new ideas. This is not the case for analytical thinkers, who may be restricted to the linear-logical path. A missing link or absent part of the network marks the dead end of the analytical process, but provides a visual thinker with a window for discovery.

Although creativity has the surface appearance of being an asset for visual people, it can present problems. The visual recall process reaches into new areas, exploring and discovering by simply looking into the mental picture of what is known. The unknown areas of the vision are simply filled in with probable entities. This process can go either way — right or wrong. When right, the visual thinker becomes a hero, a great inventor. When wrong, he has made an ass of himself.

The visual tendency to ask, "Well, what if . . . ," may be the greatest source of conflict between the two different worlds of truth.

**Timeframe.** For visual people, thoughts and words are elicited from an ongoing barrage of supporting visual mental images. Time becomes incoherent and is not a contributing factor in perception. Recent knowledge is recalled and remembered side by side with old knowledge.

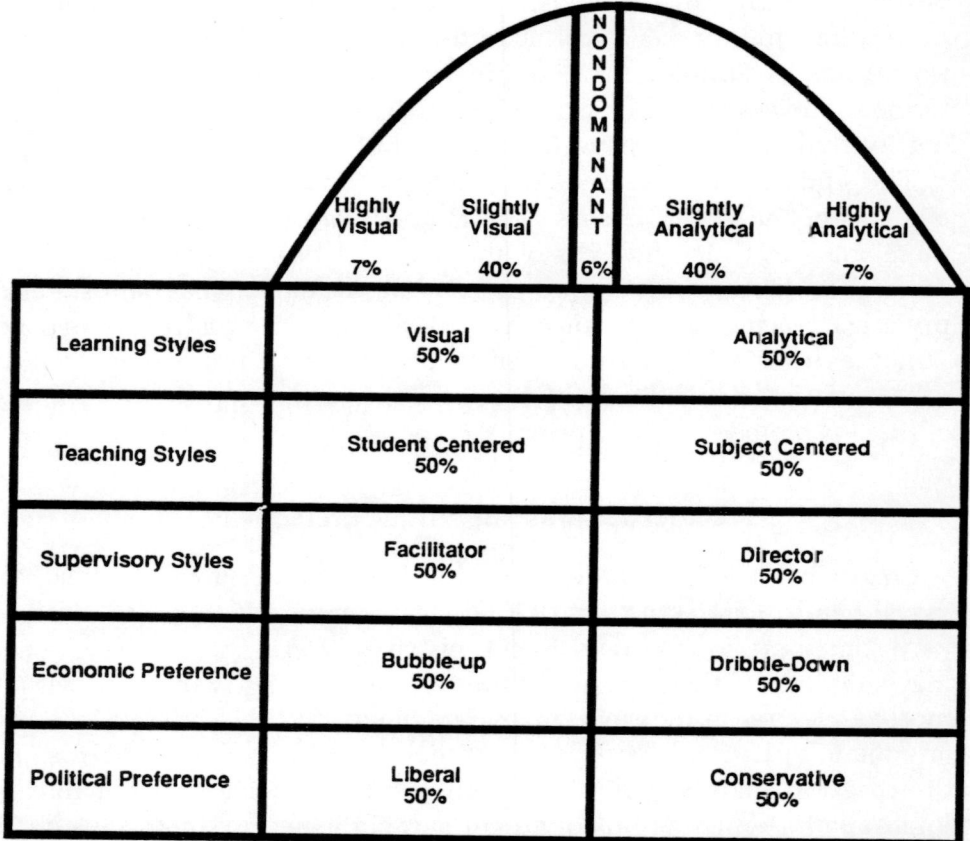

**THE HEMISPHERIC PREFERENCES OF SELECTED LIFE-STYLES**

*Figure 4.* A normal distribution of the hemispheric preference traits reveals that a majority of persons display both analytical and visual traits in different areas of their lives. The persons at or near center are likely to be indistinguishable. However, those persons further out from the center are more likely to consistently display one or the other of the two traits.

Because of this apparent incoherence of time-labeling of incoming data, presenting an oral accounting of events and experiences in a chronology is often difficult for visual people. Without a nurtured mechanism, learned to compensate for this shortcoming, many visuals can be psychologically or socially compromised by the traditional classroom, which often stresses linear-logical structures.

Sonnier relates an example of nonchronological arrangement of data.

When he was in high school in the early 1940s, he followed the *Saturday Night Hit Parade* on radio and bought the weekly magazine in which the lyrics of these popular songs were published. For many years later, he could reference events that occurred during these specific times, relating events to a particular song or its progress on the top ten list. Fixing an exact chronological date for the same incidents is almost impossible.

**Social Styles.** Visuals tend to display a more caring nature, emphasizing charity. Before the modern era of American Medical Association, some medical doctors were well-noted for charitable nature. Medical schools were admitting students by their desires and abilities in those days. By their caring nature, it is evident that some visual students became doctors. Today, there are few, if any, visually-oriented doctors because of the highly analytical admission standards to the medical schools.

**Reading.** Witelson (1977) found that a large number of dyslectic children who can read well or can't read at all had what she determined to be two visual hemispheres, rather than one each. If this is the case, then it explains why reading creates a universal problem for visual people. The mechanism of the visual hemisphere is simply just not readily equipped for the reading process. Visual people can learn to read, of course, but must often resort to a word by word approach which denies them the fluency demonstrated by analytical people.

**Admission Testing Discrimination?** One of the most problematic situations facing visual people is the lengthy entrance exam. Because of the way that visual people read, lengthy tests are merely a test of endurance and not cognition. Because visual people read one word at a time, meaning is not as directly sifted as perhaps it is for analytical people. Even after even one hour, they emerge totally sapped of energy. To force a visual person to continue for hours is a failure to understand the purpose of testing.

The way that visual persons derive meaning from text is also in need of consideration. They have instant access to more data than analytical processors may, but this same mechanism may turn against them: they may read irrelevant information into a question and formulate wrong answers.

For these reasons, rigorous testing for admission to academic, professional, or vocational programs could be seen as discriminatory practice — Sonnier would say, "Admissions testing is the analytical's way of keeping visual people out of colleges, graduate programs and medical schools."

Given the opportunity to attend, visual students can do just as well as analytical students, and perform equally well as professionals in their chosen fields. Facing lengthy and complicated admissions testing may prevent many visual people from fulfilling their potentials (see Chap. 10).

Sonnier relates this interesting footnote to visual thinking. He is in a habit of doing crossword puzzles, and recently stumped by a clue: "long-continued practice." His answer appeared, at first, to be "USE_E", but the first E should have been an A, because he had misspelled another answer, TIARA. In a dream that night, he was lecturing to a group of people on the merits of recycling. His script was written so that he could see just a few words before and after they were spoken. The word USAGE was to be said, but it was highlighted in larger letters and bold print. He awoke, got up, and went to the puzzle, fixed it, and then went back to bed and to sound sleep. He thinks that this is a rather common way that the visual hemisphere has for helping people to solve problems.

## Understanding the Analytical Preference

**Order.** The chief strength of the analytical mindset is order. Through a strict adherence to established patterns of perception and behavior, analyticals maintain the stability that people value in human institutions. Resisting the visual challenge to generate change through unconventional means, analyticals prefer to integrate new information into existing frameworks of thought. Should a ghostly apparition appear before two people, one of whom is visual and the other analytical, the visual person maybe willing to speculate the figure is indeed a visitor from the spirit world, and can entertain all manner of explanations, from the practical to the outrageous, when seeking to explain the phenomenon. The analytical individual will begin a careful, systematic approach to defining exactly which known laws can account for the effect, resisting the possibility that something "supernatural" or beyond the established concepts of nature has taken place.

This approach can backfire. While paying such careful homage to established norms, the analytical person can overlook a great number of possibilities. Science is the best example of this trend in visual thought. For centuries, the idea of spontaneous generation—living matter arising out of organic matter (eels from mud, for example)—was held to be a fact.

The first explorers who challenged that "truth" by suggesting some entirely different force was responsible were derided as madmen.

Only when a significant number of scientists codified that eels did NOT arise from mud did "truth" shift—the challenging belief became a new norm. Since most breakthroughs occur when someone manages to challenge a widely-held theory, the analytical dedication to the established and accepted can suppress the revelation of new information.

**Information Processing.** Analytical persons have a natural sense of order which affects their basic approach to information of all kinds. Unlike their highly visual counterparts, highly analytical persons will place events, incidents, and information into a rigidly maintained hierarchy. Past, present, and future are woven into strict chronological order, a progression of moments. Printed information can quickly be decoded and stored by the analytical individual, who tends to be a strong reader.

This ability to impose and respond to order is the analytical's greatest educational asset. The traditional system of education, with its emphasis on an orderly sequence of progressively complex skills, is an analytical paradise. Approaches to education which stress skill acquisition, like behavioral objectives in lesson planning, are strictly the creation of the analytical mind, breaking down broad concepts into countable, measurable, quantifiable data. Unfortunately, the analytical love of quantification and justification cannot easily deal with those subject areas which require some subjective response.

**Social Styles.** While visual persons serve a valuable function when challenging established norms of society and government, a strictly visual approach could lead to chaos. Neither preference would be served by mass instability; therefore, a system of checks and balances or a code of order is an absolute necessary. The analytical preference lends itself to the authoring of this skill of legalistic activity, creating and defining the system which creates the institutions around us.

The tidal system of HP forces acts beneficially upon social institutions. For example, analytical persons build up rigid systems of function and control and visual persons see them as barriers and seek to break them down. As systems and institutions are broken down and rebuilt over the years, the analytical contribution is stability—ensuring that, with change, total disorder does not result.

## Conclusions

An understanding of the nature and nurturing of hemispheric preference will awaken public consciousness and provide motivation for unity in all of the social institutions. Because of its all-encompassing role as the basis for all of the other institutions, education has an immediate need for this attention. With the implementation of holistic education, all of the other institutions could adjust holistically by falling into democratic alignment and pursuing the common good of both visual and analytical people.

When one source of values dominates the social process, everything goes amuck. If only visuals perform research, the rigid steps of scientific method might be neglected. If only analyticals perform research, breakthroughs from radically different approaches to old problems will become less frequent. A world of totally visual doctors could result in a loss of the systematic procedure of medicine. A world of totally analytical doctors could result in a nepotistic, clannish medical environment in which the independent thinker becomes extinct. The political arena is likewise in need of HP diversity and variety, with liberal visuals and conservative analyticals cooperating to end the name calling and to institute a democratic pursuit of the common good.

The combination of the two sources of values yields truth, which can be easily unfolded when discourse is conducted in good will. Good communication—good education—resolves the two values of truth by nurturing the perceptions which we, by nature, may be lacking. If we believe like C.S. Lewis that unity and diversity are two sides of the same coin (of humanity), then we can advocate with John F. Kennedy in his inaugural address that both sides should always explore problems that unite us rather than belabor problems that divide us.

## Chapter 6

## CONSERVATISM VS. THE "L-WORD": AN EXPLANATION OF HP IN HUMAN INSTITUTIONS

Isadore L. Sonnier[1] and James J. Asher[2]

We present an outline of the propensities of the two hemispheres with the suggestion that these are the raw materials, tools, or propensities of *the hemispheric preference phenomenon* (HP) as exhibited in the personality development of individual differences (see Figs. 5 and 6). How to communicate with each hemisphere is also presented in outlined illustration for easy reference (see Fig. 7). We also suggest that these propensities are given to each person in different and variable prescriptions from a total absence of one or the other to a generous portion of each. According to the Sonnier Model of HP, a few persons are highly visual and about the same number are highly analytical. This appears to be a normal curve distribution with most people being one or the other, but only slightly visual or analytical. These traits appear to be the raw materials for both personality development and human behavior.

A review of these contrasting works carried out by the two hemispheres leaves little doubt that the visual hemisphere is a ready and willing worker for one's personal and educational welfare, while the analytical hemisphere, it appears, may impede personal and educational success.

**Individual Differences Due to HP.** It is suggested that individual differences in thought processing modes are a function of HP, i.e., thought processing occurs either visually or analytically in most people. Furthermore, personality development in all other areas of individual difference characteristics is likewise a function of HP. The area of most common awareness of this phenomenon is the "fighting words" or "name

---

[1]After Isadore L. Sonnier (Ed.) (1989).

[2]After James J. Asher (1988).

- **It Evaluates Everything**
  Explains what's wrong
  Explains why it won't work
- **Sensitive To Flaws**
- **Is Skeptical**
- **Resists New And Untried Experiences**
- **Defends Familiar and Ordinary Circumstances**
- **Argues for Precedent to Prevail**
- **Is Gatekeeper**
- **Is Defensive**
- **May use Sarcasm, Ridicule and Rage to Vanquish "Intruding Idea"**

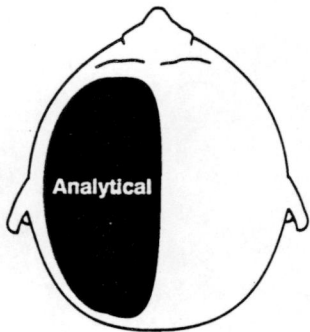

## HOW THE ANALYTICAL HEMISPERE PROCESSES INFORMATION

*Figure 5.* The analytical hemisphere is defensive, evaluative, and critical of everything, and by so doing, is a gatekeeper which resists new and untried experiences. It may use sarcasm, ridicule, and rage to keep out intruding ideas.

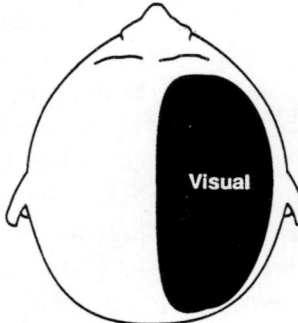

- Non-Evaluative
- Non-Judgmental
- Is Open
- Is Trusting
- Believes that anything is Possible
- Is Creative
- Thinks in Visual, Kinetic, and Auditory Images
- Thoughts are often in Code (bizarre images in night dreams)

## HOW THE VISUAL HEMISPERE PROCESSES INFORMATION

*Figure 6.* The visual hemisphere can be easily reached by bypassing the gatekeeping, analytical hemisphere. This hemisphere is not only open and trusting, but is the seat of creativity. However, without some analytical input, thoughts are distorted, as they are in dreams.

calling" between liberal and conservative social and political confrontations. However, given the understanding that these are not only real, but necessary diversities, human beings need not have destructive confronta-

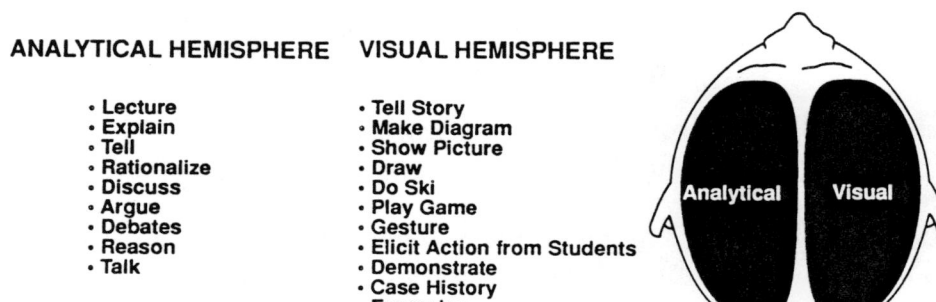

| ANALYTICAL HEMISPHERE | VISUAL HEMISPHERE |
|---|---|
| • Lecture | • Tell Story |
| • Explain | • Make Diagram |
| • Tell | • Show Picture |
| • Rationalize | • Draw |
| • Discuss | • Do Ski |
| • Argue | • Play Game |
| • Debates | • Gesture |
| • Reason | • Elicit Action from Students |
| • Talk | • Demonstrate |
|  | • Case History |
|  | • Examples |
|  | • Illustrate |

### HOW TO COMMUNICATE WITH EACH HEMISPERE

*Figure 7.* There is the need to keep a balance in communications between the two hemispheres. Once the visual processes are established, in play and game, holistic communications are established as the norm for the lesson at hand. Most of the students are reached and taught.

tions, but constructive confrontation. The fact of the matter is that these are a natural check and balance system giving assurance that all is well for the good of mankind in all social institutions.

**Who are the Liberals and the Conservatives?** According to the propensities that determine a rather large set of these HPs, liberals are nonevaluative or nonjudgemental, open, trusting, faithful to the system, and creative. The conservative's lifestyle reflects the analytical HP which analyzes and evaluates everything, is sensitive to flaws, is skeptical, resists new and untried experiences, defends familiar and ordinary circumstances, and argues for the precedent to prevail. In comparing these two extremes, it appears that the very concept of a democracy has its roots in the visual HP while clearly, dictatorship and totalitarian rule has roots in analytical, authoritarian thinking. As innocent as it may appear, any movement in the direction of nationalism is clearly a threat to the democratic forum. The liberal or visual HP lifestyle is egalitarian rather than elitist and can only breed equality and prosperity for all, in accordance with democratic principles.

**Which is Best?** In the management of social institutions, truth has two sets of values and both are needed in order to liberate its reality. One value system is not superior to the other. However, there is an atmosphere of prosperity and less elitism in the years of liberal, humanitarian leadership. Just as these conservative times are unbearable for liberal thinkers, the years of liberal control are as unbearable for conservative persons, particularly wealthy ones.

**Conservatism vs. the "L-Word".** The purpose of this chapter is to examine the role that HP exhibits in individuals who have charge of key leadership positions and to compare the public records of some of the outstanding men of our times. In politics, current trends of the Reagan-Bush years indicate analytical propensities to be in firm leadership control. For example, both of these elections to the presidency were based on a conservative lifestyle, characteristic to analytical hemisphere information processing. There was resistance to new experiences and argument for precedent to prevail. Postures were extremely defensive, even to the use of character assassination to vanquish both intruder and the intruding ideas.

An example of these contrasts is plucked for discussion. It was the Bush reference to the unthinkable, unspeakable, and unorthodox "L-word" that makes the best case and point about conservatism being a function of the analytical hemisphere, as related to the foregoing propensities. By stroke of the same words, the case is also made for the propensities of the visual hemisphere being the essence of liberalism.

With the craftsmanship of wizards, his speech writers were able to destroy any humanitarian consideration of the Willie Horton story or the Boston Harbor. The hidden factor in both of these cases is that the persons pointing the finger had an equal share in these fiascoes. However, a sufficient number of visual persons took the bait for the short time needed to destroy anything and everything liberal or humanitarian in that election. It was sorely obvious that these were not times for being nonevaluative or nonjudgmental, open, trusting, optimistic, or creative.

Because of his analytical HP behavior, George Bush will be remembered as "Wait-and-See" Bush, the president who ran the oval office, not so much from judgement calls, but by poll watching. This leadership style makes no aggressive attack on anything, unless it is to its own social, financial, or political advantage. Generally, decision making is difficult, and the record is very clear on this. The years of conservative leadership leave few agencies of the any government operating without the stain of fraud and personal use of the tax money. Yet, this get-rich-quick and rich-get-richer mentality believes the average-to-middle income worker should put stolen money back into the coffer. It is reasonably sure by any visual person's analysis of these times that future taxes will pay for this looting in both the S&L and the HUD scandals, with little retribution from the perpetrators.

During years of liberal dominance, there is widespread attention to feeding and housing the needy. Wealthy people, visual and analytical, are the keepers of these purse strings. Therefore, these are prosperous times for more people. Greed is kept in check and has less of an opportunity to flourish. However, during conservative years, elitism sets in as an acceptable standard and those in leadership roles prosper politically and financially. Wealth is accumulated in fewer and fewer hands. Companion conditions are poverty, hunger, homelessness, and diminished medical and mental health care. During conservative times, there is obvious contempt for humanitarianism and all those who practice the "L-word." The wealthy get richer and the poor get poorer.

**Unless Understood, HP Diversity Breeds Social Disorder.** While there are many other areas to use for examples, we choose politics because of its inflammatory nature. The sixties were troubling times of widened diversity between the two value systems. For conservatives, it was a time of duty to increasing nationalism. For liberals, it was a time of imposition, repression, and exploitation. The draft system was imposed by conservative force to fill a perceived Vietnam need. This was the last straw of indignation, and liberals fought back on every front that they could muster, spanning an even wider gap between the ideologies or life styles. The beauty of democratic order is maintained only when social, psychological, medical, political, economical and all other institutions are meted with liberty and justice for all.

**Other Individual Differences Due to HP.** The following chapters illustrate some individual differences due to HP. However, HP is not yet universally understood or accepted as a matter of fact. Not until then can we expect researchers even begin to study how it is nurtured. To avoid throwing the baby out with the bath water, it is pointed out that these discussions bring the real world of human behavior into clearer view. And, it is our conclusion that the HP phenomenon will soon be public knowledge with the understanding that its truth has two values and both are needed to liberate its reality. These values, and some of the solutions to problems, are discussed in subsequent chapters by different individuals who describe HP diversity in current issues.

## Chapter 7

# THE SONNIER MODEL OF EDUCATIONAL MANAGEMENT: IMPLEMENTING HOLISTIC EDUCATION

Isadore L. Sonnier and Claudine B. Sonnier

The Sonnier Model of Educational Management (SMEM) rests on the premise that hemispheric preference is the basis for individual differences among teachers and learners alike (Sonnier, 1981, 1985, 1989). The SMEM offers a way to determine the level of positive, neutral or negative affective attainment of a lesson presented, along with the level of cognitive achievement. It also offers a way to determine the degree of teaching and learning effectiveness, knowing that the level of success can be improved through holistic education strategies.

*Holistic education* is implemented when a teacher supports verbal expressions with visual aids to illustrate each point of the topic presented. Both the analytical and the visual hemispheres are reached when a topic is linear-logically presented, illustrated, and thoroughly explained. *Cognitive achievement* is enhanced because the level of teacher-effectiveness is increased. When students understand the materials and are learning effectively, *affective attainment,* pleasure in learning, generally follows.

To the question of what makes one teacher more or less effective than another, Sonnier (1989) wrote that it can be nothing more and nothing less than the teacher's ability to communite a lesson. "The process that takes place is communication. The effective teacher communicates—teaches. The ineffective teacher fails to communicate and leaves too many unanswered questions in the minds of the learners" (p. 195). Understanding the burden of communication with all of the students is the teacher's responsibility.

Unlike the use of teaching aids in the traditional sense, holistic education requires the extensive use of both visual and explanatory support so as to effectively communicate each lesson. For example, in the 1988 Warner Brothers movie *Stand and Deliver,* visual students are as effectively reached and taught as are analytical students. The SMEM offers a technique for monitoring this high level of teacher-success.

**Rationale.** Any lesson taught has but four cognitive/affective outcomes (see Fig. 8). The four categories (Sonnier, 1981) of the SMEM are:

*Category 1: Students Learned and Enjoyed the Lesson a Lot.*

*Category 2: Students Learned a Lot But Did Not Enjoy the Lesson* is acceptable to analytical teachers, who are subject-centered, but not to visual teachers, who are student- or person-centered.

*Category 3: Students Did Not Learn Much But Enjoyed the Lesson* is acceptable to visual teachers, but not to analytical teachers.

*Category 4: Students Did Not Learn Much and Did Not Enjoy the Lesson* is not an acceptable educational outcome.

| COGNITIVE ACHIEVEMENT | AFFECTIVE ATTAINMENT |
|---|---|
| 1. Students Learned a Lot | And Enjoyed the Lesson a Lot |
| 2. Students Learned a Lot | But Did Not Enjoy the Lesson |
| 3. Students Did Not Learn Much | But Enjoyed The Lesson |
| 4. Students Did Not Learn Much | And Did Not Enjoy the Lesson |

**FOUR CATEGORIES OF COGNITIVE ACHIEVEMENT / AFFECTIVE ATTAINMENT**

*Figure 8.* The effectiveness of a lesson taught can be determined by comparing the amount of cognitive achievement (the quantity learned) through the usual unit or end-of-lesson test. Affective attainment (joy in learning) can be determined by simply asking the student if they DID or DID NOT enjoy that lesson. The result provides a way to determine the appropriateness of any lesson plan and may even provide clues on how to improve its next preparation (after Sonnier, 1981).

Holistic education raises the level of teacher-effectiveness of any teacher towards the attainment of *Category 1*. The recommended standard is at least 80 percent of the student responses in *Category 1* (see Fig. 8). Grade achievement of A, B, or C is an acceptable indication that a student has "learned a lot" (see Fig. 9, Item 1).

Any lesson taught has but *three affective outcomes: POSITIVE, NEUTRAL, or NEGATIVE* (see Fig. 9, Item 3: A Lot = Positive, Some = Neutral and Very Little = Negative). Items 1 and 3 are used to determine the four cognitive/affective outcome categories (see Fig. 10).

---

Lesson _____

1. I made (or expected to make) on the tests and quizzes of this lesson:
   _____A _____B _____C _____D _____F
2. This grade is: better than _____, equal to_____, or less than_____, the amount I learned.
3. I enjoyed learning this lesson: a lot_____, some_____, very little_____.
4. The pacing of the lesson was: too fast_____, okay_____, too slow_____,
5. How could the lesson have been presented to help you learn and enjoy materials more?
Comments: _____
_____
_____

---

## STUDENT CHECKLIST FOR COGNITIVE ACHIEVEMENT / AFFECTIVE ATTAINMENT

*Figure 9.* Cognitive achievement is indicated in the first response and the level of affective attainment is indicated in the third response. Note that "enjoyed a lot" is an indication of positive affect, "enjoyed some" indicates neutral affect, and "enjoyed very little" raises the flag of negative affect (after Sonnier, 1989).

**Conclusion.** Category 1 is the only valid measure of a healthy learning environment. Although the 80 percent standard is relatively high, 90 percent is easily achieved. However, indications are that few teachers are able to sustain a level over 90 percent. Since this evaluation method is new to educators, an unsuspecting teacher could *lecture without using visual aids* and get a response-outcome from the students as low as 20 to 30 percent *Category 1* with few complaints from anyone. However, with proper concern and the use of holistic strategies, any teacher can maintain a healthy teaching/learning environment well above the standard.

Any teacher can self-evaluate cognitive/affective teacher-effectiveness by allowing the students to respond to one lesson taught traditionally

## CATEGORY 1
Lesson _____  LEARNED A LOT. ENJOYED A LOT.
1. I made (or expect to make) on the tests and quizzes of this lesson:
   XX A ____ XX B ____ XX C ____ D ____ ____ F
2. This grade is: better than ____, equal to ____, or less than ____ the amount I learned.
3. I enjoyed learning this lesson: a lot XX, some XX, very little ____.
4. The pacing of the lesson was: too fast ____.
5. How could the lesson have been presented to help you learn and enjoy materials more? _____
Comments: _____

## CATEGORY 2
Lesson _____  LEARNED A LOT. ENJOYED VERY LITTLE.
1. I made (or expect to make) on the tests and quizzes of this lesson:
   XX A ____ XX B ____ XX C ____ D ____ ____ F
2. This grade is: better than ____, equal to ____, or less than ____ the amount I learned.
3. I enjoyed learning this lesson: a lot ____, some ____, very little XX.
4. The pacing of the lesson was: too fast ____.
5. How could the lesson have been presented to help you learn and enjoy materials more? _____
Comments: _____

## CATEGORY 3
Lesson _____  LEARNED LITTLE. ENJOYED A LOT.
1. I made (or expect to make) on the tests and quizzes of this lesson:
   ____ A ____ B ____ C XX D XX F
2. This grade is: better than ____, equal to ____, or less than ____ the amount I learned.
3. I enjoyed learning this lesson: a lot XX, some XX, very little ____.
4. The pacing of the lesson was: too fast ____.
5. How could the lesson have been presented to help you learn and enjoy materials more? _____
Comments: _____

## CATEGORY 4
Lesson _____  LEARNED LITTLE. ENJOYED VERY LITTLE.
1. I made (or expect to make) on the tests and quizzes of this lesson:
   ____ A ____ B ____ C XX D XX F
2. This grade is: better than ____, equal to ____, or less than ____ the amount I learned.
3. I enjoyed learning this lesson: a lot ____, some ____, very little XX.
4. The pacing of the lesson was: too fast ____.
5. How could the lesson have been presented to help you learn and enjoy materials more? _____
Comments: _____

## FOUR CATEGORIES OF STUDENT EVALUATION OF TEACHING

*Figure 10.* Applying the assumption that the cognitive achievement of a "C" is not only an average grade, but satisfactory learning, and that the affective attainment of "enjoying some" is neutral and at least not negative affect, *Category 1* teacher effectiveness should be at least 90 percent or better for a lesson to be considered successfully taught (after Sonnier, 1989).

(Treatment A) and comparing the results with one taught holistically (Treatment B). The cognitive/affective outcomes are compared using the B–A treatment design. While positive results indicate that the holistic treatment was superior, negative results are an indication that the traditional treatment was superior (see Fig. 11). Once convinced that holistic education increases the level of communication, a teacher can maintain the 90 percent standard by periodically testing for *Category 1* (see Fig. 12).

| NAME SCHOOL | A = TRADITIONAL | | | | | | B = HOLISTIC EDUCATION | | | | | | DIFFERENCES B-A | | |
|---|---|---|---|---|---|---|---|---|---|---|---|---|---|---|---|
| | | | | | | | | | | | | | COGNITIVE | | AFFECTIVE |
| HEMIS. PREF. | COGNITIVE ACHIEVEMENT | | AFFECTIVE ATTAINMENT | | | | COGNITIVE ACHIEVEMENT | | AFFECTIVE ATTAINMENT | | | | COGNITIVE ACHIEVEMENT | | AFFECTIVE ATTAINMENT |
| HV SV ND SA HA | TOTAL | MEAN | 1 | 2 | 3 | 4 | TOTAL | MEAN | 1 | 2 | 3 | 4 | TOTAL | MEAN | FIRST CATEGORY |
| NO. OF STUDENTS: | | | | | | | | | | | | | | | |

Subject / Lesson Topic:_____

Date(s) of Administration:_____

_____ This was the same lesson taught to two different groups.

_____ This was two different lessons taught to the same group.

TOTAL = Sum of Grades ( Check one ):

_____ Student's Assumed Grades? Or,

_____ Actual Test Achievement Grades?

A+ = 5.3   B+ = 4.3   C+ = 3.3   D+ = 2.3   F = 1.0
A  = 5.0   B  = 4.0   C  = 3.0   D  = 2.0
A- = 4.7   B- = 4.7   C- = 2.7   D- = 1.7

**FORM FOR COLLECTING DATA ON
COGNITIVE ACHIEVEMENT / AFFECTIVE ATTAINMENT
TRADITIONAL TEACHING VS. HOLISTIC EDUCATION**

*Figure 11.* Following the lead of Santos Rego et al. (in Sonnier, 1989), any teacher can empirically determine the level of *Category 1* effectiveness of a lesson taught by comparing the B − A results, where A = the Traditional approach and B = the Holistic approach. The traditional approach is herein defined as the approach used prior to understanding the necessity for an extensive use of teaching aids as required by the holistic approach.

**CATEGORY:**

| NO. OF STUDENTS: | 1 | 2 | 3 | 4 |
|---|---|---|---|---|
| | | | | |
| | % | % | % | % |

Subject / Lesson Topic: _____

Date of Administration: _____

## FORM FOR THE MAINTENANCE OF COGNITIVE ACHIEVEMENT / AFFECTIVE ATTAINMENT IN CATEGORY 1

*Figure 12.* After having tested and compared the results of the traditional approach with the holistic approach, that tedious test need not be done again. A periodic testing for the level of *Category 1* teacher-effectiveness is done so as to maintain a high degree of teaching-learning success.

## Chapter 8

# HEMISPHERIC PREFERENCE IN EDUCATION

### Isadore L. Sonnier

The hemispheric preference (HP) phenomenon may be one of the most important factors to consider when seeking a better understanding of our own individual differences among ourselves as teachers and students. HP is suggested to be the basis for *holistic education,* which seeks to teach the whole person. The whole person is served when students of both hemispheric preferences are communicated with in the teaching/learning process. The strategy requires that when explaining a point, visual aids are used every step of the way. Conversely, when a visual aid is displayed, it should be thoroughly and linear-logically explained. In this context, education is synonymous with communicating both cognitive achievement and affective attainment, thereby reaching and teaching more students (Santos Rego et al., 1987).

**The HP Dichotomy in Educational Thought and Practice.** Probably the most convincing evidence pointing to relationships between the hemispheric phenomenon and its dichotomy in educational thought and practice arose from a compilation by Bogen (1975) in which he summarized the works of forty prominent authors "who have postulated two parallel 'ways of knowing' or two 'types of intelligence' or two 'cognitive styles' " (p. 25). He cited Sperry (1973), who won a Nobel Prize for work in this area:

> The main theme to emerge ... is that there appear to be two modes of thinking, verbal and nonverbal, represented rather separately in left and right hemispheres, respectively, and that our educational system, as well as science in general, tends to neglect the nonverbal form of intellect. What it comes down to is that modern society discriminates against the right hemisphere (Bogen, 1975, p. 29).

While much of the foregoing discussion was taken from the pertinent publications, *UCLA Educator* (Vol. 17, no 2, 1975) and Wittrock (1977), another publication appeared to exemplify the tenet for hemisphericity:

*Student Learning Styles and Brain Behavior* (Keefe, 1982). Briefly, the programs, instrumentation, and research of learning styles and brain research were updated and shared by representatives among researchers and practitioners in these areas. However, the applications of brain research were seldom mentioned as characteristic of or related to learning styles.

In one exception, Zenhausern (1982) reported that "neuroeducation is a term that can be applied to that aspect of education that focuses on the interaction of the brain and behavior in learning systems" (p. 192). For this contribution, he developed a questionnaire, patterned after Torrence et al. (1977), which discerns *hemispheric preference*. Dunn et al. (1977) discussed hemispheric preference as the newest element of learning styles, suggesting its importance "is likely to gain increasing attention among those who are concerned about providing maximum instructional opportunities for all" (p. 293).

**Implementing the Hemisphericity Model.** Among early implementors of the hemisphericity model in education, Spirduso (1978) is recognized for the scholarly treatment of hemispheric lateralization in compensatory and voluntary movement—a consideration for the psychomotor domain. Edward's (1979) insight in art education was significant, as judged by the substantial popular influence that was generated. Vitale (1982) implemented a thorough understanding and treatment of hemisphericity in early childhood and lower elementary education. She provided many tests for learning styles and a broad and general implementation of the hemisphericity model at these early ages. Williams (1983) should also be mentioned for a practical interpretation of hemisphericity research as it applies to teaching and learning.

**Personal Observations of Students.** Drawing from over twenty years of personal observation with college students, evidence is that hemispheric preference is a normally distributed parameter with extremely analyticals and visuals in small populations (about 7 percent each) at the two ends. The conclusion drawn is that one must examine these two extremes, highly visual and highly analytical, in order to understand this blended mixture in most people. It is also a personal observation that these extremes are the only persons that are *very sure* of their thought processing mode. Those with an eclectic blend, and with one or the other dominant, are only *reasonably sure* of their dominance. In these observations, there were a few other persons (also about 7 percent) with an apparently equal blend, and were thus interpreted to be nondominant. In support of this interpretation, they were not only *not sure*, but were simply unable to explain their thinking mode. However, when made aware of the two modes, they readily admitted to the orchestrated use of both modes.

**Personal Observations of Teachers.** Visual teachers tend to be student-centered and practice the self-directed teaching mode. In contrast, analytical teachers tend to be subject-centered and practice the authoritarian mode. Elementary school teachers tend to be predominantly (about 70 percent) visual persons while high school, subject area teachers tend to be predominantly analytical persons. However, in both cases, when holistic education is implemented, these differences melt and most students are reached and taught. The end product of holistic education is that visual learners develop analytical thought processing skills and analytical learners develop visual thought processing skills. Holistic education brings meaning and responsibility to the traditional goal of education in the United States, i.e., to educate all students.

## Conclusion

If considering *nurture*, or environmental factors that contribute to personality development and individual differences, hemisphericity is in all probability the *nature* key to understanding the apparent dichotomy of individual differences among students and teachers. The implication for this phenomenon is that truth has two sets of values and that both are needed to liberate its reality. Unfortunately, the literature appears to be flawed with misconceptions that prevent progress in either its implementation or application.

# Chapter 9

# INSTRUCTIONAL SUPERVISION FOR HOLISTIC EDUCATION

Hampton S. Williams

Holistic Education: Reaching and Teaching the Whole Child. Although the notion of teaching to the "whole child" has been idealized for a long time, the writer's feelings are that holistic education is still in its infancy as a goal of substance. However, as we learn more about individual differences in learning and teaching styles, these goals may becoming a reality. According to Sonnier, Wesselmann, and Goldsmith (1985), many educators are now recognizing that the hemispheric preference (HP) phenomenon must be a considered factor in all curriculum preparation as well as lesson planning. Hunter (1976), addressing the National Institute of Education, had these words to say about teaching to the whole child:

> Students everywhere are exerting effort to learn, but nowhere (to the writer's knowledge) are students systematically learning how to learn more efficiently and effectively. As a result, we find students routinely using assembly line learning procedures unaware that they could know their own best learning modalities, the strategies that work for them, the most productive way for them to become motivated to learn more rapidly, remember longer, and transfer that learning successfully to new situations. In short, ... students are not learning the skills to deal with the idiosyncratic dimensions of their own learning behavior (p. 5).

Hunter's statements seem to be a call for holistic education in that she stressed the need for students to know their learning styles and benefit by using them to become more academically successful.

The holistic philosophy of education, and the instructional methods that it incorporates, states the belief that student development in both cognitive achievement and affective attainment must be a considered factor when planning for instructional learning. This philosophy recognizes the importance of accounting for the students' HPs as a means of providing effective instruction. According to Sonnier (1989),

> Holistic education is a by-product of the scientific breakthrough of the mid-50's concerning human hemisphericity and lateral dominance in thinking and learning... and explains why holistic education simultaneously and concurrently stimulates the propensities of both hemispheres (p. xii).

Sonnier (1989), a leading proponent of holistic education, states that "hemisphericity is basic to holistic education—the teaching of the whole person" (p. 13). Implicit in his discussion of hemisphericity is the need for educators to give equal significance to the two functions that are served by what has now become known as visual and analytical thought processing. The central focus of holistic education, therefore, is to provide students not only with learning opportunities that match their HPs, but to also provide opportunities for them to learn how to make use of the less-dominant hemisphere of the brain.

Cognitive achievement, according to Sonnier (1989), cannot be completely assessed without considering affective outcomes. In an essay written by Sonnier, Fontecchio, and Dow (1989), they indicate that in this respect, there are but four levels of learning outcomes (see Fig. 13). These outcomes can be managed by the measurement of cognitive achievement, assessed along with affective results. Cognitive achievement can either be assessed from test scores or by asking the learner for an assumption of a grade if tested on the lesson taught. Affective attainment can only come from the consumer of this service, the students. They are simply asked if they *DID* or *DID NOT* enjoy the lesson (see Chap. 7, The Sonnier Model of Educational Management).

Harper's (1990) findings lend support to this assessment processes. Harper conducted a study that sought to ascertain if students in traditional mathematics instruction achieved differently from those students who received holistic instructional techniques in mathematics. The findings of the study, using 541 third- and fourth-grade students, indicated that not only was achievement significantly higher among the students who received the holistic treatment, the students also reported higher affective attainment, i.e., Category 1 effectiveness (pp. 37-39).

As more and more teachers and administrators learn about and subscribe to holistic education methods, it is evident that instructional supervisors must be prepared to assist in the instructional development of teaching personnel. One of the key elements to helping the beginner

| COGNITIVE ACHIEVEMENT | AFFECTIVE ATTAINMENT |
|---|---|
| 1. Students Learned a Lot | And Enjoyed the Lesson a Lot |
| 2. Students Learned a Lot | But Did Not Enjoy the Lesson |
| 3. Students Did Not Learn Much | But Enjoyed The Lesson |
| 4. Students Did Not Learn Much | And Did Not Enjoy the Lesson |

## THE FOUR CATEGORIES OF TEACHER-SUCCESS IN THE SONNIER MODEL OF EDUCATIONAL MANAGEMENT

*Figure 13.* There are but four outcomes in teacher-effectiveness in the teaching-learning process. Effectiveness at the *Category 1* level is the only acceptable degree of success according to Sonnier (see Chap. 7).

and/or the experienced teacher to master new instructional methods is adequate supervision. According to the literature, teachers welcome suggestions for instructional improvement (Harrington, 1961; Lortie, 1975, 1976; Sergiovanni, 1987). Also, indications are that teachers are more successful and have higher morale when instructional supervision is implemented as a shared responsibility (Sergiovanni, 1987; Tisher, 1979; Williams, Leonard, and Rose, 1990).

It is not this author's purpose to compare or contrast the many contemporary strategies of instructional supervision in use around the country. However, it seems necessary to take at least a brief look at a few of the dominant models in order to arrive at some conclusions regarding how supervision in an holistic education system might be developed and implemented.

**Instructional Supervision Models.** Most supervisory models fall into one or the other of two categories, product specification or process specification. Product specification, as defined by Martin and Yoder (1984), is "a supervisory system based on supervision-by-objectives" (p. 4). In this strategy, learning objectives are clearly defined and communicated to the instructional supervisor and to the students. "Because supervision-by-objectives is student-centered, emphasis is placed on the 'product' of the learning situation; i.e., what the learner can do as a result of the teaching and learning" (p. 4). An example of this model would be "Criterion-Referenced Supervision" (C–RS) (Popham, 1969) that calls for clearly written and defensible learning objectives. Teacher effectiveness under this model, is defined as the level of pupil achievement.

While C–RS does express some concern for affective student outcomes, it nevertheless cannot be used as an holistic model of instructional supervision because this model does not mandate data collection toward Category 1 level of effectiveness. It does not address HP concerns as a concept central to teaching and learning, nor does a C–RS strategy stress the need for the supervisors of instruction to know important HP information about themselves as well as about their teachers.

Process specification is defined as "a supervisory system based on management of the teacher and his/her activities. Standard procedures are prescribed for principals" (Martin and Yoder, 1984, p. 4). Being teacher-centered, this strategy places its emphasis on what the teacher does or does not do prior to and during the teaching process. An example of this model of supervision is the "Clinical Supervision Model" (CSM) (Cogan, 1973). In this model many assumptions are stated, none of which are concerned with either cognitive achievement or affective development in the teaching-learning process.

Both of these supervisory models have been criticized because they appear to cause a "mismatch" between how instructional supervision is defined by the models and how, in reality, the models are practiced. In this regard, Sergiovanni (1987) stated that:

> Dominant models of supervision and teaching emphasize uniform answers to problems, value-free strategies, separation of process from content, objectivity, and a uniform technical language stem (p. 224).

Finally, most supervisory models are undertaken in response to the many reports that come out of national government commissions (e.g., the National Commission on Excellence in Education) or private organizations (e.g., the Carnegie Foundation). Taber (1989), criticizing these reports, said that:

> Both studies fail to broaden their outlooks by considering such aspects as student attitudes, feelings, or motivations. By failing to recognize affective education as a vital force in learning, the two reports leave untapped a major resource in the total effort to improve quality education in the public schools of the United States (p. 33).

Clearly, from these discussions, if instructional supervision is to fulfill its function within a holistic education structure, some serious changes will need to be made in the existing knowledge base of supervision. For example, rethinking will be needed in the assumptions about teaching and learning, as well as the manner in which supervisory services are to be delivered.

**Instructional Supervision for Holistic Education.** Sergiovanni (1987) implied that when caught up in the language of various instructional models (e.g., teaching effectiveness, informal, direct, artistic, clinical), there is a tendency to view teaching and instructional supervision through the eyes of those models. Teachers who follow one of these instructional models will be seen as winners in the one model but losers in the others. First, and foremost, supervision of holistic education will need a "mind set" or a language which "is mind dependent in conception and mind dominant in implementation—subjective on two counts" (p. 236).

Sergiovanni (1987) strongly implied that the various models of instructional supervision act as both "windows" and "walls" (p. 227). As "windows," each model provides a specific picture, perhaps, of how it sees reality in the classroom. As "walls," however, the same models preclude viewing other realities. In other words, we see only what and how the teacher performs his/her role (CSM), or what and if the students achieve the planned learning objectives (C–RS).

The holistic model of education, while not claiming to provide a view of total classroom reality, does seem to move the "walls" further apart to permit more of the same reality or other realities to be seen. What should be the outcomes of a supervisory process that is implemented with teachers who use holistic education techniques? The holistic supervisor would want to ascertain that the materials and the methods used by the teacher would effectively reach and teach most of the children. From a commitment to extensive use of visual materials and thorough explanations, as mandated in holistic strategies, the supervisor would expect growth toward the effective use of holistic techniques and the observation that holistic education remove hemispheric preference differences among these teachers. The Sonnier Model of Educational Management (SMEM, see Chap. 7) serves these goals well. For example:

1. Analytical teachers can be expected to be effective with Category 2 students (i.e., the students learned a lot, but did not enjoy the lesson).

2. Visual teachers can be expected to be effective with Category 3 students (i.e., the students did not learn much, but did enjoy the lesson).

The use of holistic instruction effectively reaches and teaches more students towards a larger population of students in Category 1, thereby eliminating the appearance of teaching modes derived from hemispheric preference.

As a result of teachers developing in their effective use of holistic strategies, such a technique would override or remove hemispheric preference differences among their students. For example, in the movie *Stand and Deliver*, most students ended up effectively learning calculus at the highest rank of standards. When Category 1 is maintained at a high level, visual and analytical students were on common grounds of academic achievement.

**Implementing the SMEM.** Is there a place for instructional supervision within holistic instruction? The answer can be an emphatic "yes" if there is a desire for supervision. To begin the process, this writer chose to look at an existing supervisory strategy that, with some revising, might be able to meet the needs of the holistic teacher. Glickman (1990) first gave educators a glimpse of his new theory of instructional supervision in the early 1980s. "Developmental Supervision," as it is called, posits that teachers can be placed into one of four categories based on their levels of commitment and their problem-solving or abstracting abilities. Each teacher type is carefully described in behavioral terms, depending on where they are located along two dimensions (i.e., commitment and abstraction).

Glickman (1990) posits that, "we think of supervision as the glue of a successful school. Supervision is the function that draws together the discrete elements of instructional effectiveness into whole-school action" (p. 4). He also stated that supervision, to be effective, must be a function that responds to the developmental stage of teachers. Like holistic instruction, Glickman's proposition of teachers' professional development (i.e., their level of commitment and abstract thinking) implies that the supervisor, in addition to having knowledge of instructional and learning theories, needs to collect data that will identify differences among teachers so that the interactions with the teachers will be mutually beneficial.

To accommodate the differences among teachers, Glickman (1990) presents his concept of developmental supervision. Its purpose, he says, is to gradually return control of teaching to the teachers. This, he asserts, can be done by a supervisor who is skilled in techniques that will move teachers up to his/her optimal level of development. Within this conceptual discussion, he forwards several propositions that are closely allied with holistic education:

1. Supervisors cannot assume that teachers are reflective, autonomous, and responsible for their own development.
2. Supervisors will have to redefine their responsibilities—from controllers of teachers' instruction to involvers of teachers in decisions about school instruction (p. 99).

In this chapter titled, "Supervisory Behavior Continuum: Know Thyself," Glickman carefully expounds on his views of the kinds of interpersonal skills that he claims would be helpful to instructional supervisors as they take steps to facilitate the development of deeper commitment and more effective reasoning among teachers.

Several revisions are needed if Glickman's theories are to be applied to an holistic education environment. Added to the theory of teacher development should be a discussion of the HP phenomenon and its important function in explaining instructional differences among teachers and learning differences among students. Some propositions regarding the relations of teachers' levels of commitment and their levels of abstract thinking to their hemispheric preferences will need to be stated. This suggestion raises many questions that, as yet, have not been addressed in the research literature.

The discussion of interpersonal skills that might be used in developmental supervision, according to Glickman (1990), can be placed into three categories: "directive," "Collaborative," and "Nondirective." It would seem that educators acting as instructional supervisors might need to know their own hemispheric preference, to analyze that information in order to ascertain its effect on their supervisory behaviors, and, then, to relate this to the same information about teachers under their supervision. Again, this is an interesting notion that might be addressed through research efforts.

In essence, the primary suggestion that can be given to instructional supervisors who are assigned in school districts that have a stake in the success of the SMEM program is that they begin to consider the same aspects of interpersonal behavior that apply to teacher-pupil interactions as they implement strategies to supervise teachers.

What, then, are some specific assumptions about the supervision of teaching and learning that might be basic to holistic education? Conceptually, one would:

1. assume the importance of HP concepts in all teaching-learning acts;
2. assume that this knowledge of teachers' and pupils' HP is essential to effective teaching and to the achievement of cognitive and affective outcomes;
3. assume that the instructional supervisor has knowledge of his/her own HP and is sensitive to this when working with teachers who have different HPs;
4. assume that instructional supervisors are knowledgeable of the effective use of audio/visual aids, as mandated by the SMEM.

The list of assumptions is hardly complete, but it is a starting point to the development of a strategy of instructional supervision that might be more compatible with holistic education and the SMEM. From this list, however, several supervisory responsibilities can be stated. The instructional supervisor should:

1. help teachers to become aware that their own HPs affect their teaching methods.
2. help the teacher to understand that holistic education strategies may remove the need to be concerned with students' HPs in that it reaches and teaches most students effectively.

**Holistic Education Mandates Extensive Use of Visual Aids.** Sonnier and Goldsmith (1985) said that highly visual presentations stimulate learning for both visual and analytical students. According to these authors:

> ...this means simultaneous and concurrent use of models as visual aids, writing important words on the board, showing pictures and diagrams (all visual hemisphere stimuli) with simultaneous verbal expression of each concept (p. 27).

Sonnier and Kemp (1980) found that this strategy raised students' levels of achievement in both cognitive and affective domains. Finally, Sonnier (1989) stated that:

> ...all supervisor-subordinate transactions such as principal/teacher and teacher/student are heavily dependent on the former's understand-

ing of his/her own hemispheric preference and those of the subordinate for successful interaction (p. xv).

## Conclusion

The writer has attempted to determine both how an instructional supervision strategy might be compatible with holistic education and the SMEM and how such a strategy might be developed. In doing so, types of instructional supervision strategies have been identified and given brief critical analyses in regards to their possible compatibility to holistic instruction. The claim was made that Glickman's "Developmental Supervision Theory" might provide, at least, the basis for such an endeavor. It is this writer's belief that there is a place for instructional supervision within an holistic education program towards the Category 1 maintenance of the SMEM program.

## Chapter 10

# RELATIONSHIP BETWEEN HEMISPHERIC PREFERENCE AND STANDARDIZED TESTING

### Arthur R. Southerland

Educators use standardized test scores as the basis for screening and placement decisions which profoundly affect students' lives from kindergarten through professional school. Yet, few are sensitive, or apparently even alert, to the negative impact that the hemispheric preference (HP) phenomenon has on these test results for a substantial number of people. In spite of the fact that the negative outcomes of this assessment process are unintentional, there is substantial evidence that built-in bias discriminates against people with a visual HP. Consequently, these individuals are systematically screened out of programs or penalized in placement on the basis of a single, undeserved test score.

When using the results of such test scores for the purpose of screening or placement, a number of factors that contribute negatively toward success for visual persons should be taken into consideration. For example, a multiple choice test that was developed by (and for) analytical persons will contain "correct" answers which must be arrived at through linear, analytical processes. However, a visual respondent may see a different choice as the "right" answer from a holistic, inductive viewpoint. While the visual person's choice may be as reasonable as the "correct" choice, obviously a test key does not respond to rebuttal, and the response is marked "incorrect."

I am reminded of the sixth grader's response to a multiple choice item on a test that required the determination of how many miles a man could walk in 4 hours, if he walked a distance of 3 miles in one hour. When the youngster selected 9 miles as the right response instead of 12 miles, an inquiry determined that the child was aware of the right answer being 12, but had allowed time for the man to stop, look, and enjoy the scenery.

Another major factor for consideration is that visual respondents read differently than analytical respondents. Visual persons read, "word, word, word, ... " and assimilate meaning from clusters of words, a process that is tedious and tiring. Lengthy tests become a matter of physical endurance, a factor that is never considered when assessing and using test results affecting the lives of these individuals. It is important to understand the HP contributions toward the natural differences in human thought processing so as to provide all persons with an equal opportunity for success in both testing and placement.

For these reasons, it is discriminating to use the results of these test scores to bar visual persons from professional training programs, if they are so inclined. If a motivated, visual person is inclined toward entering a profession, let there be no doubt that successful and outstanding participation in that profession is in high probability. Indeed such screening selects only what Sonnier (1975, 1976) has described as "constructivity," the analytical hemisphere's phenomenon comparable to the visual hemisphere's "creativity."

Contrary to existing conditions, it would appear to be an asset to a profession to have both types of minds present to do the work and to solve the problems of the profession. Take into consideration the mind boggling problems plaguing the medical profession for having a preponderance of constructive minds, in the absence of creative minds. The problem-solving process is stifled. Simply by screening out creativity, the probability of professional mistakes and misjudgments leap well into the realm of reality. This cloud looms just as dark on university campuses with pride in admission standards that systematically exclude most creative minds that apply for admission.

Those who defend a particular test's validity and reliability are quick to point out the strong correlation between scores on standardized tests and student success in a particular program of study. However, what appears to be a valuable predictive measure for screening applicants may in more profound actuality be evidence of a closed, elitist system of constructive minds, with creative minds in absentia. It appears to be commonplace for students who score well on exams that favor the analytical HP to be admitted to programs in which they are taught by faculty members who were themselves admitted on the basis of similarly biased tests.

Furthermore, these faculty members probably have a strong tendency to use a teaching method by which analytical persons learn best. It would be expected, then, that examinations given by these teachers will produce consistently lower scores among those visual learners present who have successfully negotiated admission screening. In current practice, visual people are routinely eliminated from programs to which they have gained admission, based on incompatibility between teaching method and their learning style. Given an understanding of improved teaching methods, such as holistic education, that reach and teach both propensities, this problem can be solved by professionals. However, the worst scenario is that students are not allowed to demonstrate their abilities to learn. Left alone, the open market, pass-fail policy would be the most equitable admission policy for the good of all society.

Thus, faculty and administrators, with an analytical HP, may point to grading curves, retention rates, and graduation rates as verification for the accuracy of their admission procedures and policies. On the other hand, these highly regarded indicators of "excellence" may instead be indicators of fallacies in measuring devices and of shortcomings in the interpretation of test scores. Meanwhile, many bright, creative people are excluded or pushed out of programs for entirely wrong reasons.

Although bias against visual people is most often found in the traditional mode of content construction, it follows that the traditional mode of presentation will also take its toll. Where it is the intention of the instructor to reach and teach all students, all students learn. This was shown to be true in the calculus program presented in the book and Warner Brother's movie, Stand and Deliver. The visual learners emerged undistinguished from analytical learners. The teaching mode is holistic, i.e., reaching and teaching both propensities simultaneously, and all students participated effectively in the learning process.

Not only is there little doubt, it is common knowledge that visual people are most disadvantaged by the not-too-subtle bias that appears in the standardized tests that are used in the screening and placement processes. After the recognition of a problem, there comes the identification of solutions. Remembering that visual learners form mental pictures and do well when directions include audio-visual aids, it is easy to see that even the design of instructions on how to respond to a test may also work against these individuals. Test format and construction may be one part of this solution.

For example, if the instructions on how to proceed on an exam are given in sentence form without illustrations, visual respondents may begin such an examination with a handicap. While looking for solutions, even the testing environment should be considered. Since visual respondents are more inclined to be motivated in an environment that elicits positive affect, even the demeanor of the exam proctor may detract from their performance.

Where these differences are valued, the input of both visual and analytical realities can only bring the health and wealth of prosperity to institutional management. The question is neither whether testing should occur, nor whether there should be sorting or screening of students based upon reasonable standards. The real issues are twofold. First, both test content and administration policy must be rendered free of discrimination. Secondly, decision making for sorting and screening on the basis of test results must become more sophisticated and comprehensive commensurate with the HP phenomenon.

Considerable progress has been made in eliminating racial and cultural bias from standardized tests. So can these assessment tools be reviewed and revised in order to eliminate discrimination based on HP. Finally, educators must become more adept at interpreting test scores.

Our nation is increasingly struggling to maintain a competitive edge, a posture which requires the development of all our intellectual talent. To achieve this goal, methodical, analytical thinkers are needed. At the surface level, appearances indicate an aim toward meeting this need with intent and purpose. But deeper, there appears to be a void in meeting the need for creative thinkers. With rising entrance exam scores, where are we selecting those individuals who can stretch the parameters of perception? With the intention to weed out slow students from programs, where are we training those who can sift through what is perceived to be the logical way to do something and lead the way to innovative solutions? Just as precious metals take on strength when mixed into alloys, it is suggested that the contrasting intellectual skills of analytical constructivity and visual creativity complement each other to yield a brain trust of maximum potential.

## Chapter 11

# A BRAIN DRAIN IN
# THE ENGINEERING SCIENCES

WALTER W. FREY

I am an electrical engineer and have worked as a design and development engineer in advanced radar systems and in particle accelerators since 1957. In considering my peers over these last 30 years, I have come to the conclusion that many of them were highly visual persons, and like myself, dyslexic. I entered engineering school because I was drawn to its sciences and mechanical devices, and the study of how things work. Although unaware of it at the time, I was drawn to the engineering school's basically nonverbal courses, a selection that was strongly influenced by my dyslexia. If the United States is to advance its position in the engineering sciences, the school systems must be made aware of the problem that they have imposed on themselves by not coming to grips with the hemispheric preference (HP) phenomenon and its subsequent learning styles.

Witelson (1977) found that children with developmental dyslexia had two visual hemispheres, instead of one visual and one analytical, like most people. In that these thought processing propensities of the two hemispheres, visual and analytical, are exhibited in a mutually exclusive manner, Sonnier (1982b, 1985a, 1989) has suggested that children who enter the first grade already reading have two analytical hemispheres and that all others have blended faculties with one usually dominant over the other. He is also of the opinion that all dyslexics are highly visual, but that not all highly visual persons are necessarily dyslexic (see Chap. 3: The Sonnier Model of Hemispheric Preference).

For both misguided and unhealthy reasons, the educational systems throughout the United States have strayed from a balanced system of what Sonnier calls the two values of truth (see Chap. 3). This absence of the visual hemisphere's creative and innovative propensities, along with its flexibility in value judgement, is notably harmful to institutions at all levels. All that is left to many institutions is a cold, logical, verbal or rather inhuman system of values. In educational institutions, for example, this erosion has left us with rigid schools, established by and for analytical students.

If the schools, particularly elementary and high schools, acknowledged that these problems exist for visual students, they would have to tailor the curriculum to account for the differences in the learning process. From our vantage point, those who manage the system might have to stop substituting slick prepackaged mathematics and science "learning modules." Elementary schools (where the problems begin) are too quick to categorize students as unable to learn science and mathematics. These courses are taught and graded on a rote memory basis, since many of these teachers have little or no science or mathematics training. Or, students get brief, canned explanations from a high-quality teacher who may not be allowed to deviate from the module format. This rigidity, and the analytical educator's need to parrot answers, discourages the probing and inquiry needed by both visual and analytical students in science and mathematics. Creative thinking is neither encouraged nor rewarded.

The engineering profession in the United States is being denied potentially innovative engineers by these systems. As it is now structured, the system screens out and discourages students at elementary, secondary, and undergraduate levels who have abilities similar to those of a large number of presently practicing engineers, most of whom graduated before 1960. That innovative group, trained on vacuum tube technology, developed semiconductor electronics and computers, lasers, optical communications, satellite communications, AND put a man on the moon. I believe that a significant portion of these engineers are highly visual and dyslexics.

Dyslexics often resist admitting that they are afflicted, in part because the public equates dyslexia with lack of intelligence. The engineer who has worked hard to get a degree and advance in the profession fears the return of feelings of inadequacy and stupidity usually experienced during earlier school years. A feeling of "sneaking through" the system is common. Once the dyslexic acknowledges the problem, however, and reads more about it, he or she can begin to cope with resentment and anger and deal more effectively with feelings of low self-esteem that may still exist.

The thinking processes of visual people, especially dyslexics, do not mesh well with the established learning process. However, I am sure that some make it. To resolve the conflict and keep up, they must invent novel learning processes. They hone these processes until they have converted what many would consider a handicap into an asset. Albert Einstein is but one example of those who become engineers and scientists and go on to develop creative and innovative ways of storing information and making connections. However, analytically oriented entrance exams to programs are eliminating the creative potential of professions and institutions alike (see Chap. 10: Relationship Between HP and Standardized Testing).

Before there can be a solution, there must be the recognition of a problem. Highly visual and dyslexic children will have to be identified at an early age. The literature on dyslexia highlights the extreme cases, which are generally recognized in early school years. But mild dyslexics must compensate on their own. Teased as slow learners, late bloomers, or lazy students, mild dyslexics respond with anger toward the school system because they know the material but cannot respond as quickly as their peers.

Here are a few of my suggestions for solutions:

1. Screening for and keeping highly visual and dyslexic tots in the mainstream of education is so important, because nature is in place. But, with appropriate nurturing, they are the cream of the crop.

2. By the time the students enter college, such screening could identify potentially intuitive and innovative engineers.

3. At earlier schooling level, only high-quality teachers should teach math and science in order to give students a firm foundation on which to build advanced concepts. Extensive use of practical examples should be made so as to enhance knowledge and utility of mathematics in science.

4. Colleges must also stop using foreign-born teaching assistants who speak English poorly and put these classrooms back into the hands of full professors who have more extensive knowledge and experiences. The heavy accents and lack of fluency result in the student only understanding every third or fourth word, a severe handicap to a struggling visual student.

To the question of what makes one course more affectively influential than another, Sonnier (1989, pp. 195–196) wrote:

> It is always the teacher. It can only be the teacher. It can never be anything more or less than the teacher. And, the only logic that I can place on the process is that of communications. The effective teacher

communicates—teaches. The ineffective teacher fails to communicate and leaves too many unanswered questions in the minds of the learners. Step-by-step communication, with visual aids... *HOLISTIC STRATEGIES* beget *NOT ONLY* a higher degree of achievement, they beget affective results! (See how to obtain and to maintain this level of communications through The Sonnier Model of Educational Management, Chap. 7.)

5. There must also be more communication between academia and practicing engineers.

6. The school systems must adjust their curricula to reflect the basic knowledge needed by engineers in their everyday work.

Unfortunately, too many companies and laboratories will only hire graduates with a B or better grade-point average, which is no indication of an engineer's ingenuity. These potential employers should instead keep an open mind about visual and dyslexic students, who could fill positions where their innovative and intuitive approaches to problems could be utilized. I think it is because they had to depend more on input from peers to get through school. Generally, I have found that the "C" student is more of a team player.

Like Sonnier, I believe that although on most critical issues the proponents must come to an agreement to disagree, truth has two values, visual and analytical, and that both are needed to keep our institutions afloat with reality (see Chap. 3). A conservative, analytical leadership that systematically excludes and condemns liberal, visual thought and input is more and more the rule today, rather than the exception. Such leadership and such a system can only go amuck for lack of innovation and creativity.

## Chapter 12

# HEMISPHERIC PREFERENCE AMONG SCIENTISTS

Isadore L. Sonnier

Analytical values in science are a powerful source of truth. However, if the Sonnier Model of HP is considered, as in all other institutional enterprises, analytical values supply science with partial truths. The visual values have played a more important role in science that has been credited. Both visual and analytical values are needed to liberate scientific truth.

A good example of this is that for years, one could read about solar prominences at one location in a textbook and sunspots were located elsewhere. The truth of the matter is that prominences and sunspots are the result of a magnetic storm within the sun that shoots out a torrent of magnetically repelled gases at one location and magnetically attracts the torrent back to the sun at another location, thousands of miles apart. When the sun is eclipsed by the moon, the torrent can be observed on the outer edge of the sun and the event shows up as solar flares, or prominences. However, when the same event is observed on the surface of the sun, the torrents of gases are sufficiently cooled to shadow the radiating gases and each flare is seen in pairs as dark sunspots.

It appears to be difficult for analytical perception to make the connection that these are one and the same phenomenon. However, this is typically an observation that can easily be visually perceived and connected as one and the same phenomenon.

Photography, a two-dimensional representation of three-dimensional phenomena, plays a significant role in scientific investigations. However, as in the prominence-sunspot investigations, in which photography played a significant role in data gathering, this is a tool that has almost exclusive utility for visual scientists. For example, an atmospheric electricity teacher, one of the early photographers of lightning, left little doubt about being a highly analytical person because of what appeared to be an inability to visualize the 3-D reality of his 2-D photographs.

He was a master teacher because he used these visual aids in sufficient quantity and quality to be called an holistic educator. His illustrated lectures were not only interesting to his students, they all appeared to get deeply involved in the presentations. He was excited about an ongoing investigation of the distribution of light on some particular slides that he had taken of bolts of lightning. He had discerned *areas of greatest and least concentration of light,* graphically illustrated by curves of intensity distribution.

The only problem with this, and the two publications generated by these investigations, is that one cannot reduce a 3-D phenomenon, like lightning, into a 2-D model or representation for the purpose of studying the original phenomenon in 3-D. Once reduced to 2-D, depth no longer exists as a dimension and one cannot determine anything of scientific value about the original, 3-D event. The distribution of light on the slide could not describe the 3-D event as he was doing it.

In yet another example of photography to make the point that analytical scientists have a weakness, if not an inability, to accurately observe visual phenomenon. In many of the books on lightning, there is one photograph that is referred to as "beaded lightning." It was obviously valued by a number of authors who used it as an illustration in their lightning books. It shows a stroke of lightning on a radio tower at the summit of a mountain. It is branched across the entire visible sky of the picture. The unique thing about this photograph is the large number of beads that pock the lightning event. For this reason, it is called "beaded lightning" with little or no attempt to explain this strange lightning behavior. The partial truth of the matter is that it was accepted and displayed as just that, a phenomenon of lightning.

The other value of this truth can be visually perceived as a photographic phenomenon. The camera was focused on a point in a distant plane, being the radio tower on the mountain. The event took place roughly across the plane of the focus. The beads that show up on the film mark an event of lightning that is either coming towards the camera or going away from it. As it streaked across the focus, beads showed up on the film that cannot be distinguished as going toward or away from the camera. Even if one was to try to make this distinction by identifying the first one as towards or away, there is no way to discern this. With the rather thick focus planes of today's lens, it is conceivable to have two beads created by two rather shallow successions in the same direction, say, one towards the camera and the next one towards the camera, again.

Usually, *science and technology* are not perceived as an HP-related phenomenon. However, when the differences and merits are discussed by a visual and an analytical person as science vs. technology, the two values of truth promptly emerge. Many who call themselves scientists are really science educators or technologists. Scientists are those visionaries and creative people who contribute to the body of knowledge. According to the SMHP, analytical persons dabble somewhere in the scientific enterprise in what they consider to be a rather static body of knowledge. Being analytical does not preclude pioneering in the unknown and contributing to the body of knowledge. However, it is more likely that those ready and willing to alter the scientific body of knowledge are visual people.

My hope is that science educators throughout the spectrum of the scientific enterprise, including medicine, will stop assuming that analytical values are the only source of truth and come to the realization that truth has two values and that both are needed. Entrance examinations to college science departments serve only to magnify problems that riddle professions throughout the scientific enterprise. Another area for concern is in the evaluation of fundable research projects by fund granting agencies, public and private. For starters, how can new, different, and innovative projects be discerned if fundable projects are limited to areas within the body of knowledge? How can innovations be funded if the evaluator requires a sound and hard fast area of knowledge in which to innovate? The use of a grantee's track record for "satisfactorily" having dispensed with funds in the past is too often used as a source of trust that he/she will continue to "satisfactorily dispense" new funds that are granted. The absence of visionaries in this area, among grantors and grantees, is not difficult to detect.

## Chapter 13

# HEMISPHERIC PREFERENCE AS A FACTOR IN PUBLIC POLICY FORMULATION

### G. Richard Larkin

After twenty years of close contact with British career civil servants, Snow (1961) wrote a glowing review of their intelligence, honorableness, toughness, tolerance, generosity, and mastery for the short-term solution. Snow was impressed with how they forcibly conduct their business with no fuss and a dash of intellectual sophistication; however, he expressed concern over their lack of foresight.

Snow's concern for the lack of foresight among men in government has been and continues to be echoed by observers of public affairs in the United States. George Will (1983) states, "I tremble for my country when I think that schools may be sending forth into government people who are too proudly 'practical' to take ideas seriously. Although God . . . knows, such 'practical' people have government pretty much to themselves these days" (p.. 16).

Senator Daniel Patrick Moynihan (1981) offers evidence to support the concerns of Snow and Will. He states that in Cabinet or the Sub-Cabinet service under four presidents, there was never " . . . a serious discussion of political ideas—one concerned with how men, rather than markets, behave. These are necessary first questions of government" (103).

The men that Snow, Will, and Moynihan describe possess many of the characteristics and methods of operation associated with what Sonnier (see Chap. 3) describes as analytical hemispheric preference (HP). According to this model, the analytical HP tends to view the world as complete and fixed for eternity and emphasizes maintenance of the status quo. People with a visual HP tend to view the world as dynamic and evolving and emphasize responsibility and action that befit changing times.

Sonnier contends that political views are heavily influenced by HP. People with an analytical HP tend to be conservative and people with a visual HP tend to be liberal. He contends that over representation of either one of these HP modes in government is unhealthy. "No institution can survive, nor the society that condones it, without the democratizing touch of both liberal and conservative input" (see Chap. 6).

In recent times, government dominated by a conservative force has led to less than optimal results in Democratic and Republican administrations and in foreign and domestic policy formulation. The problem is like a two-sided coin. Seeing just one side at a time leaves one in conceptual absence of the whole coin. My objective is to describe these two sides as separate forces of light, with both being viable forces of institutional support. They are, however, antagonistic forces by nature and therefore in need of informed, democratic supervision.

**Foreign Policy.** No man in government in recent years has embodied the analytical HP more staunchly than Robert McNamara. Halberstam (1969) provides an excellent illustration of this point. He describes McNamara as a tense and driven body with a mathematical, analytical mind. He could bring order out of chaos and had the ability to support his rational position with statistics. Everyone was impressed with McNamara, if not in awe, in fear. "For [his] was a mind that could continue to summon its own mathematical kind of sanity into bureaucratic battle, long after the others, the good liberal social scientists . . . had trailed off into dust" (pp. 217–218). Even when the sanity of his mathematical version did not work out, in the light of profound failure and down to the ebb of his tenure as Secretary of Defense, even then, he never abandoned his faith in rationality. His rationale was that he regarded Vietnam as a failure because it was no longer cost-effective (pp. 217–218).

McNamara's public policy formulation, in dealing with Vietnam, epitomizes one of the United States' great foreign policy failures. From an analytical rational perspective, these policies should have worked. However, what this mode of thought processing fails to take into account is that many people do not view the world from an analytical perspective. The visual images of the human-cost of the war, flashing across the television screen every evening at the dinner hour, had a powerful impact on a disgruntled population of Americans with a visual HP. Public support for the war policy polarized the people for and against it. Today, it is clear that such a one-sided, analytical-conservative formulation was likely to fail because it lacked the moderating effect of visual-liberal input. The United States is still suffering from the repercussions of this policy failure.

**Domestic Policy.** One of the most frequently debated issues in domestic economic policy is whether or not the federal government should provide subsidies to influence location of economic activities. The debate generally centers around equity-efficiency tradeoffs and represents a classic example of how political attitudes may be influenced by HP in policy formulation, analyticals being the conservative force and visuals being the liberal force.

Levy (1991) describes the equity-efficiency dichotomy in terms of industrial location. If a site is the most efficient location for a firm, ordinary market forces will lead the firm to that site. Levy cites as an example, "If a subsidy (say, in the form of an industrial park site delivered at a fraction of actual cost) is necessary to cause the firm to locate there, by definition, the site is not the most efficient location. Thus, following this logic, there is a loss of efficiency for the whole economy stemming from the use of subsidies to influence economic locations" (p. 207). Such a choice is less than efficient because of the cost of producing a certain type of good or service would be greater than if the firm made a location decision without the benefit of a subsidy. An example of an efficiency-equity tradeoff is to oppose public intervention in favor of economic efficiency. To lend the powerful support of public intervention is to favor equity. In general, the visually-oriented liberals tend to favor place-related programs. Analytically-oriented conservatives tend to oppose such programs, arguing that it is the government's role to provide conditions for business success, but not to intervene in decisions on how or where capital should be invested.

During the past decade the conservative efficiency view has prevailed. Because of the difficulty in identifying the long-term effect from these few short years, the results of the total dominance of one point of view have been mixed. From the rational, analytical perspective, the policy has been a success. Inflation and interest rates have remained low and growth in employment and GNP have been steady. From a visual, liberal, and more humanistic perspective, the results are remarkably different. According to Reich (1991), after accounting for inflation, the wages of two-thirds of all workers are 16 percent below what they were in 1973. Since 1989 three million American children have fallen below the poverty level, 1.2 million Americans have lost their homes, and the infant mortality rate has increased by 2 percent. Another alarming fact that threatens the very core of traditional America is income inequity has increased to its highest point in 40 years with the top 20 percent of the work force earning more than the remaining 80 percent.

## Conclusion

Sonnier argues that an important conclusion can be drawn from the theory that individual differences are due to HP. Truth has two sets of values and both are needed to liberate its reality in the management of human institutions. In these examples of public policy formulation which I have presented, only one set of values was considered. The results are less than satisfactory for the public interest. These examples appear to substantiate the need for the democratizing input of values from both forces to maintain policy formulation and institutional management that has promotion of the public interest as its major objective.

## Chapter 14

## HEMISPHERIC PREFERENCE IN THE RISE AND FALL OF A BUSINESS

WILLIAM C. SMITH

The formula for a successful business venture boils down to a match between the firm's offering, its product or service, and the market that its founder has decided to serve. For innovative products, this product-market match usually results from an entrepreneur with a large imagination, coupled with determination, timing, and luck. The ability to be successful in the birth and operations of a thriving business enterprise has much in common with the effective management of other social institutions. As such, it provides an excellent opportunity to examine the input of the different hemispheric preferences (HPs) in business management from birth, through the day-to-day operations and decision-making processes, and in the evolution most businesses generally go through.

Going by Sonnier's assumption that very few people have use of both analytical and visual propensities in a nondominant manner (see Chap. 3), most people are to some degree either visual or analytical. Looking at the two basic natures of HP, it is fair to presume that new product-market matches come more naturally from persons with a visually dominant HP. If this is true, then new businesses are most likely to be founded by visual people rather than by analytical people.

People with an analytical HP are risk-averse. They prefer to analyze all the details and find it difficult to take the leap of faith, from idea to conceptualization and implementation, necessary to start a business. While analytical persons tend to gather as much data as possible, they also tend to "wait and see" and to "examine all sides of the issue" before they make a decision. "I'll move on that idea as soon as everything is right," is a commonly expressed precaution. On the other hand, visual persons generally feel more comfortable with the risk and ambiguity inherent in any new venture.

However, a successful business requires more than just a start. As it grows and develops a routine, management becomes more and more focused on this routine and establishes rules and procedures so as to ensure every customer with the same quality of service or product. It is in this internal management capacity that the analytical persons play a major role in business success. They are adept at developing rules and procedures, with flow charts, necessary to maintain control of the enterprise as it grows.

Externally, if the market being served were a static phenomenon, all businesses would continue to be successful. But, the marketplace is a dynamic phenomenon, always changing and moving. Some markets, for example, microcomputers, move at a blinding speed. What was a very successful product-market match in the past may lose its future because consumers suddenly begin to demand something new. To ensure success, any business must constantly renew itself, both internally and externally, by adapting its product-market or service offering to match where the market is at any given time.

In order to meet all of these pressures and demands on a business, there is the need for input from both visual and analytical people in order to keep all sides of ongoing issues grinding in the decision-making process. For example, arguments that may appear to be counterproductive to one side, visual or analytical, may well be the input required to meet the customers' changing needs, adapt to the changing environment, internal and/or external, and to continue to operate profitably.

The following scenario displays what can be characterized as the typical pattern in the evolution of a business toward (1) stagnation or (2) continued growth and success:

1. A business is created in the mind of an entrepreneur and becomes a reality through his/her ability to get others to buy into this vision.

2. The product-market match envisioned is realized when sales begin to grow. More employees are added to handle the increased demand.

3. Customers want products that better match their individual needs and begin to make peripheral demands. To meet these demands, product/service offerings are expanded. Competitors enter the market with imitations or an improved way to meet the need identified by the innovating entrepreneur. The innovator either (1) becomes defensive and protects the "established" product/service, or (2) meets the competition head-on by using or improving on the product/service.

4. As growth continues, facilities are expanded and more employees with various specialties are hired. Management's attention is focused on policies and procedures to CONTROL the enterprise. (1) The need for operational control of the enterprise supplants sensitivity to the marketplace as management's top priority. Or, (2) sensitivity to the marketplace remains management's top priority.

5. As long as the product-market match remains in place, the firm prospers, even if overly focused on an efficient operation. However, consumer-needs being dynamic, (1) a static organization, focused on a particular product/service, can not survive. (2) remain attuned to the market and change offerings to fit customer demands.

It appears to be that as the market changes, rare is the management that can maintain sensitivity to that marketplace. For most businesses, the very structure needed to control the organization, its personnel, assets, and vested interest in established policy and practice, may actually impede growth and profit. As the administrative organization grows, so does the apparent need for analytical input. Attention is overly focused inward, leading to more and more bureaucratic formalities. Failure is on the horizon when external change is resisted in favor of administrative convenience.

The alternative is to maintain channels of input from both sources, internally from employees and externally from customers. In order to preserve the vitality of a business, a balance must be struck between the outward focus of maintaining a product-market match while at the same time inwardly focusing on the freedom of input and communications throughout the operation of the enterprise. Going into new territories for the business, based on employee suggestions and customer-requests, appears to require input from people with a visually dominant HP. The policies and practice of the operational care of an existing business appears to require the input of people with an analytical HP.

With vision there is the potential for recognizing a product-market match and some sustaining growth and development. However, there is less of a potential for overseeing and the coddling of established territory as is possible for analytical people. On the other hand, an analytical person, or even the brainstorming results of several analytical persons, can only lead to the conservative building of a fortress around their business. What is perceived as appropriate nurturing may indeed be the tightening of a stranglehold.

If these assumptions are true, then for a business to be successful, people with both HPs must be allowed to contribute freely to the firm's policies and product/service directions. During these times of nervous economic fluctuation, when managers face novel situations to which past experience is nonexistent, it may be wise to seek input from different people with these different values.

Companies like IBM, Hewlett Packard, and 3M may be examples of management that have successfully blended the need for people with both HPs. With this in mind, a knowledge of how HP influences the decision-making processes in entrepreneurship, as a social institution, appears to be in need of further study and may have a niche in both, the art/science of marketing and in marketing education.

## Chapter 15

# HEMISPHERIC PREFERENCE IN MORAL THEOLOGY

### Isadore L. Sonnier

It is neither by accident nor by chance that among Christians, hemispheric preference (HP) plays a decisive role in the process of making moral decisions. Christian thought is herein explored. However, the same discourse could describe any of the major world religions, because the reason for diversity is so basic as to be part and parcel of the human nature of HP. Some of us process our thoughts with a visual HP, others with an analytical HP, resulting in two different sets of overt personal traits (see Chap. 3). It is with this basic assumption that Christian personal and interpersonal behaviors are reverently discussed.

How does a Christian make moral decisions? How should a Christian make moral decisions? To these questions, Bosnick (1990) said that among Christians of today, we find three avenues of thought. One is the Evangelical Protestant position, holding the belief that all answers are found in the Bible which is seen as the sole source of authority for Christians. Even among these, individuals migrate to the two basic sides. Those who take the conservative view resist change, especially deviation from the Protestant tradition. The liberal position is that change is needed and they offer lots of it, but usually come up short of what they had in mind. Year after year, often at the annual convention, each side is poised to counter the movements of the other side, only to end up with moderates at the helm. These moderates are usually individuals who have gained at least a limited trust from both sides.

Among other scholarly Christians, a rather comparable scenario is played. Bosnick (1990) described the second avenue of moral decision making to be conservatively based on the authority of the Catholic Church, as expressed by either the Magisterium, or that found in tradition and time-tested values. He described the third avenue of Christian thought to be a liberal position which emphasizes the right of each individual to follow their own personal consciences.

Bosnick (1990) stated further that the contributory elements to Christian decision-making can be subdivided into those external to the believer, scripture, tradition, and the Magisterium; and those which are internal to the believer which include, virtue, reason, and conscience. It appears that in all of Christendom, advocates of traditional values are brought into conflict and must struggle with the advocates of change. Liberals express both want and need to change many things and conservatives are entrenched with intent and purpose to allow no change.

It is suggested that HP is the undercurrent structure of diversity and the driving force among both leaders and followers. It is the agent of cohesiveness that bonds individuals to one side or the other. In compliance with this theory of HP, conservative individuals tend to reflect the analytical hemisphere's propensities. They analyze and evaluate everything, are sensitive to flaws, are skeptical and defensive, tend to resist new and untried experiences, defend the familiar and ordinary circumstances, and argue for the precedent to prevail. On the other hand, liberal individuals tend to reflect the visual hemisphere's propensities. They are nonevaluative or nonjudgemental, are open, and are trusting. They show faith in the system, and are creative (see Chap. 6).

One system is not superior to the other, but each one needs the other for the mutual benefit of common cause. Sometimes, in debate, points of agreement are so scarce that one must be forged in the interest of common cause and mutual benefit of all that are affected by a decision. As with the other lores and areas of institutional management that are described elsewhere, application of the HP phenomenon to the processes of moral decision making compares very well. Separately, visual and analytical values are inadequate on their own, even though each exposes and expresses important values of truth. It is proposed that the ultimate source of these values flows from the individual differences of HP. Analytical individuals take the conservative path to derive values of reality while visual individuals take the liberal path and the two seldom meet. If this is the case, then truth has two sets of values and both are needed to liberate its reality.

The iconoclast controversy serves to show HP in an historical perspective. For nearly the first thousand years of its history, Christianity wrestled with the theology of the use of icons in its liturgy. Both visual and analytical artists undoubtedly took a guarded stance against the making and veneration of portraits of Christ, the saints, and landmark events. Iconophyles used these as visual aids to teach largely illiterate congregations. The principal objection offered by iconoclasts was the Old Testament prohibition in the Second Commandment concerning the veneration of false gods. There was also the fear of violating Christ's divinity and/or humanity.

The iconophyle view eventually gained theological approval with the view that veneration of icons was on the symbolic nature of the image, and that it served as a prototype for whom the veneration was addressed. The fact that these arguments linger serves to place the controversy squarely as an HP values conflict. Analyticals support iconoclast values while visuals support iconophyle values. To this day, these values are in conflict and they continue to surface and evolve.

Among many others, HP issues that are in current debate include *clerical celibacy, sexuality, abortion,* and *the use of extraordinary means to extend life.* These debates immediately draw into battle, not so much the moderates, but the extremes of both sides. Each side predictably explains what is perceived to be "the answer"; when in reality, the morally "correct" answer may lie in the amalgamated values of both sides.

Gula (1989) described these structures as time-valued and as moving from structures of the past, the "classicist worldview," to the contemporary, "modern worldview." The structures are herein suggested to be "analytical" and "visual" views in a timeless constant. People have always engaged in debate over values that issue from HP differences (see Fig. 14).

Given the process of debate, a fully Christian position acknowledges not only the importance of scripture, church tradition, the church's teaching office (Magisterium), and conscience, but also adds formation in wisdom and other virtues. Views that are limited to only one of these elements do Christian morality a disservice and make it more difficult for intelligent people to respect Christian moral positions (Bosnick, 1989).

The conclusion is that when issues are managed by the monologues of extremes, settlement is kept out of reach, even for the moderating effect of eclectic input. However, truth can be resolved only with fair and honest representation from all concerned, mutual respect for different HPs, and with disagreement as an acceptable point of departure. To-

| FEATURES | ANALYTICAL | VISUAL |
|---|---|---|
| CHARACTERISTICS | Views the world as complete and fixed for eternity. | Views a dynamic and evolving world through historical development. |
| | The world is marked by harmony of an objective order. | The world is marked by progressive growth and change. |
| | Speaks of the world in terms of well-defined essences using abstract, universal terms. | Speaks of the world in terms of individual traits using concrete historical concepts. |
| METHOD OF OPERATION | Begins with the abstract and derives principles from universal essence. | Begins with experience and derives accumulated experience. |
| | Deals with universals of humanhood by deriving principles from the physical nature of being human. | Deals eith the historical person in historically particular circumstances |
| | Conforms to authority and to pre-established norms. | Formulations of norms are historically conditioned |
| | Emphasis on duty and obligation to reproduce established order. | Emphasis on responsibility and actions fitting to changing times. |
| | Primarily deductive. | Primary inductive. |
| | Conclusions will remain the same. | Some conclusions will change as emperical evidence changes |
| | Conclusions are always secure as long as deductive logic is correct. | Leaving room for incompleteness, possible error, open to revision; conclusions are as accurate as evidence will allow, but these are accurate enough. |
| ADVANTAGES | Clear, simple, and sure on views of reality an conclusions about what to do. | Respects the uniquesness of the person and the peculiarities of historical circumstances |
| DISADVANTAGES | Tends to be authoritarian in the sense of claimimg to have answers suitable for all times. | Tends to be relative in the sense that everything is conditioned. |
| | Tends to be dogmatic in the sense of having the last word. | Tends to be antinomian in the sense that all laws are relative. |

## THE UNIVERSAL VIEWS RESULTING FROM VISUAL AND ANALYICAL THOUGHT PROCESSING

*Figure 14.* Visual and analytical HPs can be clearly delineated as the basis for the chemistry of group dynamics. The two different hemispheres generate mutually exclusive, universal views that in turn reflect their respective sources in document production. For example, analytical people tend to formulate conservative documents while visual people tend to formulate liberally-oriented documents. However, given the benefit of values input from both views, the product will in different degrees and in various ways be of greater benefit to all concerned (adapted from Gula, 1989, pp. 32–33).

gether, visuals and analyticals have the potential to dialogue a refined path through mutual cause, towards the attainment of common benefits. Could it be that both *the process* and *the emerging truth*, described and herein attributed to HP, are how the "Mystical Body of Christ" works among the people of God?

## Chapter 16

## HEMISPHERIC PREFERENCE AND CRIME

Thomas R. Panko

Incarceration is a common means of attempting human behavior modification in the criminal justice system. Euphemistically, this behavior modification is referred to as "corrections." In instances where a rehabilitation-oriented system has been institutionalized, the sentencing of individuals to public service/vocational rehabilitation is often used as corrective measure. However, where little distinction is made concerning the nature of a crime or between types of criminals, incarceration becomes the popular mode of correction. In this scenario, there are few offense-specific rehabilitation programs.

Individuals who advocate a system which features a staircasing of programs upward from reprimand, restitution, and public service to incarceration as a means of behavior modification, are aligned with Sonnier's definition of visual HP (see Chap. 3). In the field of criminal justice, truth seems to have two orientations: the people-oriented "visuals" and the law-and-order-oriented "analyticals." Visual people take the stance that human beings have within themselves both the need and desire to function successfully within society. On this side of truth, given the right match with an appropriate program, few prisoners need to be incarcerated. An alternative would be to sentence an offender to perform public service in order to enhance both self-esteem and respect.

"Analyticals" vigorously disagree with this strategem and view crime and criminals in Manichean terms. In this view, breaking the law results from a conscious decision to cross over to the wrong side of social order, even though this behavior may be related more to situational conditions. The staircase of programs advocated is a set of punishments scaled to different crimes. Thus, a satisfactory criminal sanction is associated with a given number of years of incarcerative punishment; some crimes entail more years, others fewer years of punishment. (And, sometimes the sentences are virtually indistinguishable.) In this perspective, with each draconian sentence a message is conveyed to all other would-be criminals. Punishment is also viewed as deterrent, a means of crime prevention. It is designed to discourage others from stepping over to the wrong side of the law. This is the most commonly expressed need for institutionalizing the death penalty at the extreme end of the punishment continuum.

At the expense of overstatement, the utility of capital punishment as a criminal sanction is basic to HP. Given the variables associated with one's nurturing, the "visual person" is generally people-oriented and harbors strong feelings against the institutionalized killing of human beings for any reason. Persons with an analytical HP are more apt to advocate the death penalty because of the perceived ultimate "deterrent" message it sends to would be criminals. These are the two HP sides of the issues and arguments concerning behavior modification and criminal justice.

Existing research and personal observation underscore the fact that a substantial population of inmates are nonreaders, school dropouts, and lacking in social and vocational skills. Perhaps this is a subtle indication that most inmates are visual people. If so, this may mean that visuals are more likely to be apprehended, sentenced, and incarcerated precisely because they are visual. The fact that many prisoners are vocally expressive and mirror the profile of a "con artist" suggests that their traits may well be more visual than analytical. The flip side of these values is that analyticals dot every "i" and cross every "t" of the law, even to obey every traffic signal, suggests that the crimes that they commit are of the white collar nature with a milder penal code.

It appears that visual offenders are people who have slipped through the cracks of the educational institution. If this assumption is correct, then we know that this can be rectified. That we can reach and teach more of the visual students throughout the educational enterprise seems a highly tenable proposition (see Chap. 7). If the assumption is correct that analyticals tend to be the white collar offenders and have a milder penal code for themselves, then this too has a solution. If truth has two values and both are needed to liberate its reality, then input is needed from both sides so as to eliminate dual standards.

Another observation relates to the people working in law enforcement. Institutional mismanagement occurs when police/prison guards over time must deal with crime and criminals to the extent that they come to despise both crime and criminals. Thus, it becomes progressively easier for them to abuse anyone perceived as a criminal. To wit, the "keepers" themselves exhibit the brutality of the "kept."

The recent incident of alleged brutality by officers of the Los Angeles Police Department will not only be on our minds, but will haunt police departments everywhere for a long time to come. Other than the consideration that the analytical HP is less capable of humane discretion than the people-oriented visual HP, my impression is that this has little, if anything, to do with HP and more to do with inhuman, mob, or animal instinct. It serves as a reminder to all about "the fundamental nature of the law and law enforcement." Lawmen are not "the law," but should be trained and skilled in "enforcement of the law." How to avoid breaking the law in the name of law enforcement is an ever present concern that should be given curriculum priority in skill development for rookies, as well as inservice and continuing education programs throughout the institution.

Another source of institutional mismanagement issues from the assumption that institutional managers, operators, or administrators are somehow different from the masses and must be treated differently. Dual standards clearly exist when the financier of a drug operation (a respected citizen, businessman, or school board member) receives a mild sentence to be served in minimum security institution while his two street peddlers are severely sentenced in maximum security. This white collar vs. blue collar dilemma is all too commonplace and appears to stem from HP differences.

Until now, the only solution to these arguments has been "to agree to disagree," put the issue to popular vote, and then accept and portray the resulting decision as reflecting the will of the people. It is suggested that knowledge and understanding of these HP differences will decrease the insistance that one side or the other holds the only truth, and that the respective proponents will come to realize they possess only one side of truth. With the understanding that individuals have little control over their inherited HP, disagreement with a handshake is likely to occur. In conjunction, they can create programs of dual utility at both ends of the criminal justice continuum: prevention, as well as programs that positively promote behavior modification and assist all individuals toward socially acceptable rehabilitation.

# Chapter 17

# HEMISPHERIC PREFERENCE AMONG ATHLETIC ADMINISTRATORS

### W. Harvey Poole, III

Most of the people in athletic administration, herein referred to as coaches, fall somewhere between the two stereotypes, autocratic-authoritarian and democratic-egalitarian. Since most coaches display the full range of these characteristics, the assumption is that most of them orchestrate a blend of these two extremes and are eclectic. Indeed, most do not regularly display the traits of one or the other, but of both characteristics. However, there are those who tend to display one or the other set of these traits with unmistakable regularity. Assuming that hemispheric preference is the primary cause of this behavior, autocratic-authoritarian individuals are dominantly analytical and democratic-egalitarian individuals are dominantly visual.

While some of the individual differences herein described are rather pronounced, neither set of traits is better or worse than, or superior or inferior to the other. It is only that they are different with unmistakable regularity. Selected coaches and managers who display the traits of one hemispheric preference or the other are the subject of these discussions. Although these outstanding persons tend to fully live up to the definitions of one or the other traits, they are believed to exemplify the thesis that hemispheric preference is in evidence throughout the institution of athletic administration.

## AUTOCRATIC-AUTHORITARIAN-TASK-ORIENTED

Coaches who display the autocratic, authoritarian, task-oriented traits are guided by their analytical hemispheric preference. The authoritarian coach tends toward behaviors that are very structured with emphasis on accomplishing a task (like winning a game) within that structure. The satisfactory completion of the task is his number one concern, while the establishment and maintenance of personal and interpersonal relationships is secondary.

The pattern of leadership for this coach is to establish prescribed behaviors that include rigid discipline and the punishment of disobeyers or deviators. He insists on doing things according to his beliefs and is the sole judge on how tasks are to be performed. He emphasizes structure in performance, believing that people must be coerced, controlled, directed, and even threatened in order to make them perform to his satisfaction. He believes that the average player wants to be led and avoids personal responsibility. With these personal traits, he works best with submissive assistant coaches.

This coach is rigid about schedules and plans. His behavior is formal, rather than informal, and very organized and well-planned. He may not be always right, *but* he is never wrong. In competition, he focuses exclusively on winning, makes and announces all decisions, structures the pattern of work procedures himself, and is not prone to deviate from original plans.

The authoritarian coach does not engage in coach-athlete interactions because he does not usually have a warm personality. This makes him distant or detached, and not particularly happy or friendly. He is not bothered by being disliked or even feared. His no-nonsense attitude about getting the job done tends to make him impatient with players and subordinate coaches, alike. He can often be cruel, insulting, and even sadistic.

He is task-motivated and achievement-oriented with great confidence in himself because he knows that he can get the job done. He is impervious to criticism and never doubts his own actions in the pursuit of accomplishing the task at hand. Some of his miscellaneous traits can be listed as: high need for control, "hard-nosed," often religious and moralistic, power-authority-dominance-oriented, issues orders, and is not receptive to ideas generated by others. He is often perceived as guarded, tense, disagreeable, and unpleasant.

Many of these athletic administrators and coaches go down in the history of their teams or organizations as the greatest that ever was. Some of these include Mike Ditka (Chicago Bear, football coach), Bobby Knight (Indiana University, basketball coach), Frank Kush (Arizona State University, football coach), Vince Lombardi (Green Bay Packers, football coach), Billy Martin (New York Yankee, baseball manager), and George Steinbrenner (New York Yankee, owner).

## DEMOCRATIC-EGALITARIAN-RELATIONSHIP-MOTIVATED

Coaches who display the democratic, egalitarian, and relationship-motivated traits are guided by their visual hemispheric preference. The democratic coach tends toward behaviors that are oriented toward maintaining good relationships. He is concerned with the interpersonal relationships between himself and his players. Successful achievement of the task is often secondary to the achievement of good coach-athlete relationships. He acknowledges and appreciates good performance, even when the task has not been achieved successfully.

Concerning the establishment of positive relationships, he believes in good player-player and coach-player relationships. To this end, his players can exercise a certain amount of self-direction and self-control in the accomplishment of objectives to which they are committed. He not only believes that the average player accepts and seeks responsibility, but is open to their suggestions. He encourages assistant coaches to participate in planning, seeks and expects independent thinking, and is open to their suggestions.

The democratic coach is flexible, amenable to change, willing to try something different, somewhat loose in organization, allows team members and assistant coaches discourse in both task and social interactions, and allows players to function within limits. His humanistic tendencies make him paternalistic, sincere and considerate, harmonious and agreeable, friendly, likable, warm, relaxed, and pleasant. He tries to avoid conflict, is sensitive to the feelings of others, and shows respect and mutual trust for others.

A democratic coach will be communicative, patient, and supportive. He shows care and affection for others, and does not believe in "winning at all cost," or "winning is all," or "if you don't win then you are a loser."

Many of these athletic administrators and coaches go down in the history of their teams or organizations as the greatest that ever was. Some of these include Bobby Bowden (Florida State University, football coach), Lou Holtz (Notre Dame, football coach), Tommy LaSorta (Los Angeles Dodgers, baseball manager), Joe Paterno (Pennsylvania State University, football coach), and Casey Stengal (New York Yankee, baseball manager).

## Chapter 18

# HEMISPHERIC PREFERENCE IN MILITARY LEADERSHIP

DAVID L. SONNIER

Effective leadership in all branches of the military is of the utmost importance because the stakes are so high. A failed military operation is different from a lost football game. There is no recognition of the fact that the leader of a failed operation may have had good interpersonal relationships with his soldiers, an effective leadership style, or even good sportsmanship. Therefore, military leadership must be viewed in a slightly different context than athletic, political, or corporate leadership. It is within that context that I explore and discuss the hemispheric preferences (HP) of leadership among military figures.

Military history shows many examples of effective leadership styles, each of which is different from the next. Although there appear to be as many examples of styles of effective military leadership as there are examples of effective military leaders, their HPs are discernible. For different, yet obvious reasons, leadership training at military training centers in recent years has focused on bringing out the inherent abilities in the individual without regard to HP. Even though this phenomenon is hardly even acknowledged, the readings used in various military training centers draw from the experiences of historical figures whose leadership styles could be classified as falling into one of the two categories of dominantly visual or dominantly analytical.

This recognition that there is no "rubber stamp" formula to being an effective leader is a healthy acknowledgment of the fact that it takes both types of leadership for the military, as well as any other organization of people, to function effectively. The existing philosophy, therefore, is a good one. Each and every officer, officer candidate, and noncommissioned officer going through training is to be considered a future successful leader. To expand upon this point, I draw from the leadership styles of noted historical military leaders, both of whom are frequently the topic of discussion and the centerpieces of required reading in the Army's officer training centers. General George Patton and Colonel Joshua Chamberlain were two military leaders whose different leadership styles can be compared and contrasted to illustrate the point.

Colonel Joshua L. Chamberlain was a professor at Bowdoin College less than a year prior to the critical Civil War battle at Gettysburg. Although he had no military training or experience prior to the Civil War, he joined the Army for patriotic reasons, was given a commission, and eventually commanded a Maine regiment because of his education and prestige. What he lacked in military training and experience, he made up for by studying tactics late into the evenings during the first few months of his service.

Just prior to the Battle of Gettysburg, a group of 120 mutineers from another Maine regiment were brought to him for disciplinary action. They were half-starved, convinced that their enlistment had expired and that they were only required to serve two, not three, years, and sick of a war that they thought was over and lost. It was widely accepted that the Union Army was rapidly losing the war.

Chamberlain was not only told that he could execute the mutineers, but was advised to do so before they caused more problems. Instead, he told the guards to leave, had a cow butchered, listened to their grievances, and while they ate he promised to look into the matter about their enlistment when he had time. He desperately needed these men to fill out his own regiment, which was almost as small as the group of mutineers. He offered to give back their weapons if they would join with him and fight the Confederates. All but six of them agreed to do so.

That remarkable act of persuasion and patience, in itself, was not as noteworthy as what soon followed. During the Battle of Gettysburg, the 20th Maine held the left end of the Union line, which had to be protected at all cost in order to prevent the entire Union defense from being flanked. Holding the position over two days required his stretching the line thin to the breaking point. At one point, Chamberlain had to fill a dangerous gap in the line by sending his own younger brother to defend the position. In desperation, he quickly invented a new tactical maneuver for a situation not covered in the manuals that he had studied. When the ammunition ran out, he ordered a bayonet charge. This confused the Confederates, threw them into panic, and caused them to withdraw. This victory saved the Union flank from the superior Confederate force and would not have been possible without the mutineers augmenting the force.

But more important, this turn of events was made possible by Chamberlain's improvised and creative leadership. He was recognized with the Medal of Honor and an eventual promotion to Major General. As is often the case with heroic leaders, after the war he was so popular as to be elected governor of Maine three times. What would have happened had he executed the mutineers from his home state?

Chamberlain's leadership style could be classified as dominantly visual. His approach to motivating and inspiring is "people-oriented," which is typical for visual HP. Another indication of visual HP is his ability to create and implement a new, untried, untested tactical maneuver in the heat of battle.

Contrast this leadership style with that of General George S. Patton, Jr., of World War II fame. He was a career military officer who spent his entire lifetime in training to lead men into combat. His knowledge of military history was so thorough that he believed himself to have been reincarnated. He thought he had actually participated in major battles fought thousands of years before he was born. On more than one occasion, he amazed people with his ability to walk the grounds of ancient, long forgotten battles, and describe exactly what happened, moment by moment, every square foot of ground. But through this knowledge of history, and how leaders of combat forces typically behaved under certain circumstances, he was able to read and even predict his opponents' decisions and respond accordingly.

Patton gave the appearance of having little patience with human frailty, as displayed through cowardice. He expected his men to fear him, but despite his harsh leadership style, he was greatly admired and his soldiers had unshakable confidence and trust in him. He was authoritarian and a strict disciplinarian. Because he expected the impossible of his men, he often obtained it. He blitzed through enemy territory with astonishing speed. The long-term results of his tactics were always low casualty counts and American lives saved. For example, to relieve the surrounded 101st Infantry Division, he volunteered to pull his Third Army out of one battle, move over 100 miles on no sleep and little resupply, to go right into a major engagement within 48 hours. This type of movement, with so many troops, was something never before attempted in military history, and quite impossible as far as many were concerned. What made this operation possible, in Patton's expressed opinion, was that his men feared him more than they feared the Germans. He expected his men to do the impossible and pushed them beyond the limits of exhaustion, because to the men in the surrounded 101st Infantry, the urgency of the situation demanded it.

Patton, with his harsh leadership style and vast knowledge of his trade, and Chamberlain, with his gentle persuasion and ability to use a few choice words at the right moment, provide good examples of how the two different HPs can cause combat leaders to handle situations differently. The authoritarian leadership style of Patton is indicative of an analytical HP. Key to his success was a vast knowledge of military history. It appears that he had cataloged in his mind in-depth knowledge of enemy tactics and commanders. With respect to his decision making, it appears in retrospect that his decisions were based not so much on new ideas, but on the application of old ideas, proven successful in the past. This is not to say that Patton was without vision; the opposite is true. He had vision, as a young officer, to see the future importance of tanks. As a general, he saw the future threat posed by the Soviet Union. Throughout his career, he studied the Germans that he would eventually meet in combat. Still, he provides a good example of leadership style based on a dominantly analytical HP, even though probably only moderately analytical as opposed to highly so. Given the understanding of the phenomenon's blended middle, this would account for his generous portion of visual perception.

Both of these officers are often presented as "role models" in leadership training, although they are completely different if considered in terms of what their HPs probably were. What is important is that they were both the right person for the job that they had to do in their time, and they provide the case-in-point that it takes both types of leaders in the military, as it does in all other walks of life.

## Chapter 19

# HEMISPHERIC PREFERENCE IN PHOTOJOURNALISM EDUCATION

Eddy L. Wheeler

The students who enroll in my beginner's photojournalism class have a wide range of prior knowledge and experience. In every class there are both visual and analytical students. Visual students are predisposed with a good perspective and come up with visually sound pictures because it is instinctive to their nature. However, they generally come to the course lacking in compositional rules and the ability to fuse the art and science of photojournalism. Analytical persons, on the other hand, have an instinctive feeling for compositional rules, the symbolic structures of the appropriate arts and sciences. However, they require assistance with the visualization of a good subject.

My experience is that few of these students know which they are, and it is a waste of time to try to make such identifications. By nature of these differences, each requires a different set of instructions. However, their nurturing has a way of garbling this up so that there is no pattern to the kind of help any student will need. Their personal experiences with actual photographing or with experiences leading to feelings for "the perfect picture" comes into play. Depending on their predisposition to taking good pictures, these considerations are best avoided. Some think and express the belief that they can take good pictures, while others not only display little interest, they are quite sure that they can't learn to "see" the picture ahead of time.

With this in mind, I have worked out a curriculum that takes students where they are at this point in time of their lives. The major tenet I get across is that pictures are made in the brain even before the camera is picked up. Whether the student is visual or analytical, my objective is for him or her to "see" the picture and then to snap it. I have to believe that anyone can make good pictures. Although I understand that visual students are innately gifted, they can fall prey to certain pitfalls.

I also know that analytical students do not innately possess this gift and it may be a bit difficult to acquire. I think that visual awareness is a gift that we all possess, if not by nature, by nurture. We either refine it or we ignore it. The potential is in all of us to make good pictures.

Just as it is not fruitful to wonder which students are by nature visual or analytical, it is not prudent to evaluate the hows and whys of each student's previous experiences (their nurturing). These individual differences become the very fabric of the group dynamics that contribute to this class being different than any before them or any to come after them. My concern is to pick each individual up where he/she is in personal development and to go from there.

The way that I do this is to provide all of the students with three objective experiences, allowing for their individuality to surface. Keeping in mind that there are misconceptions to be corrected and insights to flourish, the first of three objectives I have for beginners is to *study the masters*. It is not luck when Michael Jordan scores 40 points in a play-off basketball game. It's *art*. It was not luck when Eugene Smith photographed *The Country Doctor* essay in *Life Magazine*. These are examples of masters at work. They practice previsualization. There is nothing magic or mysterious about it. They simply put in a lot of time and effort in prior planning with the necessary skills to make their plans work when needed.

As with these masters, each student is to train at rapid decision making. Previsualization is the end product of this training. In photojournalism, there is seldom, if ever, a second chance. Once that fleeting millisecond is gone, it is gone forever. That experience, that feeling when everything is just right cannot and should not be rewritten, painted over, edited out, or added to in the darkroom.

The second objective that I require of the beginners in my care is *understanding the compositional rules*. The student is assisted in preplanning and previsualizing patterns of culture, then waiting for that moment, that mood, that light when everything comes together for an instant in time.

The third objective for beginning students is that of *blending art and science*. If they don't already, I help them to know their equipment so well that they can trust and use the technical and scientific aspects of it automatically. With each added competency comes joy and pleasure of accomplishment. Although each student is different, some skills come easier for visual students while others come easier for analytical students. For example, previsualization requires abstract thinking, a natural for analytical students and an acquired skill for visual students. All are potentially capable of mastering both the science and the art of photojournalism.

Some of the minor course objectives include practicing the technique of seeing, just as intently and with the same passion and concentration as any NFL quarterback practices his passing. He goes through the motions over and over again to get the timing down just right to complete a pass, the perfect pass, the one that wins the game.

Previsualization demands abstract thinking. What is often confused with daydraming is previsualization. Shooting the perfect picture means being able to stand in one spot yet walk around the subject to get the best angle of light with consideration for both the foreground and the background. Knowing which lens to use is also a part of previsualization.

Can one picture tell the story or will several shots be needed to convey the event? Will silhouette or timed exposure be needed in this visual communication? When and how to use stop action, pan or blur technique to best show motion is not as much a skill as an art form. This thinking or choosing must be done prior to the action and is at the heart of one's previsualization skills—an indication of one's status as an artist.

Because of the fact that all beginners come to this lore with different experiences and skills that stem from both their nature and their nurturing, it is not necessary to waste time, thought, and energy wondering which student is visual and which is analytical. But, with caring and patient prodding and tutoring on my part, as well as from peers, most of them perform at an acceptable level, or at least are headed in that direction at the end of the course. My job as a visual arts educator is making visual students more astute in the symbolisms of photojournalism while on the other hand making analytical students more instinctively visual.

# Chapter 20

# HEMISPHERIC PREFERENCE AWARENESS IN PUBLIC EDUCATION

Martha J. Larkin

Teaching is a demanding profession that provides the range from rewarding experiences to stressful situations. The teacher's main purpose is to help students learn and use their abilities to maximum potential. This must be done within a prescribed time period and in a designated manner. The teachers who have a visual hemispheric preference (HP) find creativity stifled in order to meet deadlines and document student skill mastery in a predetermined manner. Yet creativity is still recognized as important in the educational process, so these teachers find opportunities for creative expression rewarding for themselves and for their students. The teachers who have an analytical HP find it easy to be organized, meet deadlines, and document skill mastery. But, it may be stressful for these teachers to plan and incorporate creative experiences into the learning process. Thus, the teaching profession provides varied boundaries of pleasure and stress for teachers with different HPs.

A teacher's relationships with administrators, colleagues, and students are also associated with a range of experiences from reward and pleasure to stressful conditions. Unfortunately, many of the problems stem from lack of understanding and accommodation for HP. My comments pertain to some of the stressful problems in the teaching profession and suggestions for their improvement through a better understanding of the HP phenomenon.

**Teacher-Administrator Relationship.** Principals and the curriculum or content area supervisor are the teacher's most frequent administrative contacts. The principal's or supervisor's main task in the teacher-administrator relationship is to make certain that the teacher is performing his/her duties according to state and local policies. Because of validated instruments, teacher evaluation may have become easier for analytical principals and supervisors. With the increased emphasis on teacher accountability and effectiveness, some assessment instruments used in the teacher evaluation process tend to be more accommodating for the analytical HP. These assessment instruments allow the evaluator to determine if a particular teaching skill was observed during each teacher evaluation. On the other hand, administrators with visual HP may prefer to evaluate the teacher without documenting the presence of each skill, but rather to observe the humane processes of effective teaching and learning. For example, a high level of cognitive achievement may be gained while at the same time maintaining positive affective attainment (see Chap. 7). Although the assessment instruments commonly used today are valid and reliable, they may be easier for analytical rather than visual administrators to use. Teacher evaluation with these instruments could be stressful for visual administrators.

Visual teachers may find the results of an evaluation, done with an analytical assessment instrument, equally frustrating. When the evaluation is completed, the teacher receives a copy of the form used to document the evaluation. The teacher can determine if he/she has received at least a minimum score on each of the designated skills. The principal or supervisor discusses the results of the evaluation with the teacher. The visual teacher views the discussion with the evaluator to be more helpful than a form with numbers. This is especially true if the evaluator can describe the teacher's performance as a whole. The analytical teacher finds more merit in the documented results of the evaluation. Individual components of a teacher's performance can be isolated as teacher strengths or targeted as needing improvement. Such a performance evaluation is stressful for most teachers. The unilateral nature of an analytical instrument, used as the solitary mode of teaching assessment, creates added stress for most visual teachers, as well as for some of the analytical teachers. This factor may taint both results and justifications for the use of this method of assessment.

Teachers look to administrators for guidance. The analytical administrator is organized, adheres strictly to deadlines, and usually has authoritarian advice for most situations. The analytical teacher may find some comfort in knowing that he/she can get a definitive answer to a question. On the other hand, visual teachers feel that a decision is made or an answer is formulated by the administrator without sufficient input from the teachers. Visual teachers also find it frustrating if they miss a simple "report" deadline and for that, get a reprimand for their "teaching performance" from an analytical administrator.

The analytical administrator's organization is evident during faculty meetings. Both analytical and visual teachers seem to appreciate the organization, for example, a typed agenda for each teacher. Such organization and attention to details keep the faculty meeting running smoothly and quickly. This administrator, however, tends to issue staff reprimands, rather than to discuss misdeeds with the appropriate or responsible individuals. Visual teachers may feel that some of the topics at faculty meetings are approached in an isolated manner. Their comments reflect the belief that topics should be viewed as a part of the total picture. Sometimes analytical administrators and visual teachers find this a source of conflict.

**Teacher-Teacher Relationship.** The teaching profession attracts a large number of visual persons. Their creativity is evident in bulletin boards and room decorations, as well as daily lessons and activities planned for students. Such creative endeavors are time consuming. So keeping an organized room and completing the required paperwork on time can be difficult for these teachers. Analytical teachers may compliment visual teachers for the clever bulletin boards, while in silence, they wonder how anyone could function in such an unorganized classroom. The visual teacher may praise an analytical colleague's organizational talents which are evident in a neat and orderly classroom and well kept records, but, he/she may feel that the analytical colleague could spend more time on creative projects to enhance learning for the students.

Visual teachers frequently use available time after school or during breaks to discuss ideas and problems. This is a need which must be fulfilled even if it means spending more time at home grading papers and record keeping. Analytical teachers spend some time exchanging ideas and sharing problems with colleagues, but they tend to excuse themselves to return to organizing their rooms or grading papers. However, because of HP differences, analytical teachers are viewed as unsociable by their visual colleagues.

A conflict is evident when visual and analytic teachers are required to work on a project or paperwork which must be done in a prescribed time and manner. When the visual teacher assists with data collection, the analytical teacher often becomes frustrated when the data is collected and analyzed in a disorganized way. He/She also becomes frustrated when the visual teacher does not proceed as rapidly or as methodically as possible with the data collection and deadlines are missed. At this point, the frustrated analytical teacher wishes to take over the project in order to get it completed. This may leave the visual teacher with the mixed feelings of frustration, inadequacy, and remorse.

**Teacher-Student Relationship.** The word teacher does not adequately reflect all of the duties that are required of someone in that profession. In addition to teaching, one must also assume the duties of a secretary, disciplinarian, counselor, parent, and custodian. With all these responsibilities, it is obvious why a teacher would appreciate those students who try to do their best work and cause minimal problems. After an extremely challenging day, the teacher has little tolerance for a student who does not share the same HP. For example, the analytical teacher assists a visual student with an assignment. Once the student understands the concept of the lesson, he/she may suggests a more creative approach to completing the assignment or additional creative enrichment activities. The analytical teacher feels that the assignment must be completed instantly and there is no time for creative diversions. Thus, the teacher is unhappy when the student does not do his/her best and the student is unhappy when the teacher does not accept his/her suggestions.

The visual teacher spends time with students helping them to think through problems and ideas and looks for different approaches to problem solving. This is fun for visual students, but may frustrate analytical students who ask only, what needs to be done for a grade, when is the deadline, and please, which is the right approach to solving this problem? In mutual frustration, the visual teacher then believes the analytical student has missed the point of the lesson because of the view that there are different approaches to the solution of most problems and no one way can be isolated as the right way.

It is not unusual for visual teachers to remove themselves from any and all remnants of the "authority figure." The desk may be thought of as a symbol of authority and be placed in the back of the room, rather than in the front.

**The Special Education Teacher.** As a special education teacher, I feel the need to add these comments. I sense that a majority of special education teachers have a visual HP. Both groups of HP special education teachers face similar problems as those discussed above. Teacher-administrator, teacher-teacher, and teacher-student relationships are basically the same as for other teachers.

Special education teachers, however, have an advantage in teacher-student relationships over regular education teachers. Students referred for special education are given several kinds of tests to see if they qualify for admission to the program. A student's learning style may be determined during or following testing. This could give a clue as to his/her HP. Since special education students receive an individualized educational plan, this information is considered when his/her curriculum is planned. Thus, a special education teacher may be more aware of each child's learning style and HP. Many special education students are visual and holistic education is a viable solution to reaching and teaching these students. It is also to our advantage that special education classes are smaller than regular education classes and to the student's advantage that we can spend more time towards meeting their needs.

## Conclusion

A number of stressful problems in the teaching profession are needlessly due to a lack of awareness of HP and/or the lack of its accommodation. Stress can be reduced for teachers, administrators, and students through this awareness and its accommodation. Some of my suggestions are:

1. Implement holistic education to remove HP differences among teachers and to reach and teach more students in spite of their HP differences.
2. Include topics on HP for teacher and administrator staff development with the understanding that it is acceptable to disagree.
3. Provide brainstorming opportunities on HP for teachers and administrators. Each HP group can suggest ways that one can be more tolerant and accepting of the other group.
4. Provide opportunities for teacher sharing sessions. Each HP group can learn how to be more accepting of students with opposite HPs. Teachers can relate specific examples for sharing.
5. Explain to students that people learn and perceive differently and that it is acceptable to be different.
6. Acknowledge HP as an asset in the decision-making process.
7. Explore a new meaning for "teaching students HOW to think." They already know how to think—some visually and others analytically. What we can do is teach visual children to be more analytical and analytical children to be more visual (e.g., both objectives are included in a single math lesson).

The teaching profession holds one set of values for those with visual HP and another set of values for those with analytical HP. Both sets of values are equally important to the teaching profession. There should be a time and place for input of the values of both groups. Often, in reality, this is not the case. But, by permitting and encouraging both sets of values to flourish at all levels of education, teaching will become more successful and less stressful. This is consistent with Sonnier's position that the truth is comprised of two sets of values and both are needed to liberate its reality.

# Chapter 21

# HEMISPHERIC PREFERENCE AS A FACTOR IN STRESS MANAGEMENT AMONG NURSES

### Jean A. Haspeslagh

Nursing is a profession that often places its practitioners in a double bind. On one hand, it demands of nurses a high degree of accuracy with compulsive attention to detail and time. These are traits that are characteristic of the analytical individual, who copes well with these demands. On the other hand, nursing also demands that its practitioners be attentive to patients' psychosocial, emotional, and nonphysical needs, as well as the physical needs, typically visual traits which the visual nurse handles with ease. The double bind occurs when the nurse is faced with stresses associated with being either a predominantly visual person in a predominantly analytical system or a predominantly analytical person encountering predominantly visual demands.

According to the Sonnier Model of Hemispheric Preference (HP, see Chap. 3), most people display one or the other of the characteristics and fall prey to one or the other stressful demands. If this is the case, than an understanding of HP differences among human beings may help to resolve at least some of the problems that plague nurses to the point of stress. One can easily imagine that the mix-matching of two HP extremes on the same floor and/or shift can create a workplace stress that with knowledge and understanding of HP could be avoided or at least decreased.

Other areas where knowledge and understanding of HP can serve as a factor in stress management for nurses include the problems associated with teacher-student, nurse-supervisor, and nurse-patient relationships. It is suggested that when problems created by HP differences are perceived as natural and normal, they do not need to breed difficulty to the point of major stress. For those who wish to deal with these problems head on, the following are suggested ways to cope with the stress.

**Teacher-Student.** Some nursing teachers are easily identified by both, their demeanor and their delivery of the curriculum, as being either analytical or visual. The analytical teacher is cause-and-effect-oriented and paints a picture of nursing activities with the neat constants of a cut and dry world. Lecture is the preferred method of imparting knowledge, with content delivered in a linear-logical manner. The teacher expounds on how this begets that, or how A always precedes B.

For the visual teacher, the world is less absolute. This instructor leans toward classroom discussion, experiential activities, and away from the the strictly lecture format. The focus is more on generality with reference to global concerns and the teacher finds it difficult to quantify things. The real world is perceived and described as complex, which makes it difficult to pin things down with accurate numbers.

From the student's point of view, visual students do better with a visual teacher while analytical students prefer analytical teachers. The reason for these preferences are evident when one examines the difficulties that arise in some learning situations. For example, visual students have problems in courses taught by analytical teachers who lecture without the benefit of visual aids, rely too much on a heavy reading, and prefer to remain rather impersonal and aloof. Analytical students do well in these courses.

Because visual people tend to see the big picture of an idea, this teacher tends to paint first one section of the picture, then another, and another in a global fashion. For many of the students, both visual and analytical, this is perceived as rambling and disjointed, resulting in frustration and stress.

Recognizing oneself as being basically visual or basically analytical is the first step in remedying the stress associated with conflicting HPs in the classroom. Holistic strategies are the recommended solution for the reaching and teaching of more students at both extremes (Sonnier, 1982a, 1985, 1989, see Chap. 7).

**Nurse-Patient.** The analytical nurse is a stickler for accuracy and detail and is time-oriented. There is just so much time for this, that, or the other. The visual nurse, being more people-oriented, is in tune with psychosocial concerns, like patient feelings of comfort or discomfort, emotional needs, and the nonphysical environment. Nurse-patient relations splashes over into other areas. As can be expected, because of these radical differences in environmental concerns, nurse-supervisor relations are affected and run either smoothly or stormy.

**Nurse-Supervisor.** Nurse-supervisor relations, with a mix-match of opposite HP extremes, could be stormy because perceived needs and emphases are drawn from radically different values. "See if Mr. J. is emotionally ready for the operation but hurry because in two minutes Mr. B. needs to receive his preoperation medication." "Why are you spending so much time with Mr. S. (whose wife is an invalid at home), when you still have patients who need their bed linen changed before lunch?" These comments create stressful times for visual nurses.

In order to provide safe care to large numbers of individuals, the planning, coordination, and service delivery are set up in a manner that appeals to the analytical individual who is comfortable with deadlines and details. As a result, one finds that more successful supervisors and nurse managers tend to be analytical. For these nurses, dealing with the emotional and psychosocial demands is their nemesis. "If we didn't have to deal with all of the emotional ups and downs, we could get our work done in half the time." Of course, what one finds is a well run and efficient unit that, should the staff be predominantly visual, has a high turnover in staff. Or, a staff that feels frustrated because they went into nursing to "care" for people and not to "nurse the desk" and deal with all of the bureaucratic demands.

**Coping With Stress: Understanding HP.** Because of HP differences among human beings, the world takes on two sets of values, one for visual persons and a different one for analytical persons. It is futile to expect a visual nurse to be anything more or less than super-concerned for the psychosocial needs of patients. Analytical nurses should not be expected to be anything else than what they are, either. If the HP phemenon were understood early in their education, each nurse could improve effectiveness in their area of weakness. However, one has to be aware of a problem before the problem can be solved.

Knowledge of HP should also improve planning. Recognition of the different strengths of analytical and visual nurses, when planning and making assignments, could result in less stress for all concerned. Placing nurses in situations where they can best apply their HPs will not only decrease stress, but should also improve student, patient, and staff satisfaction, as well.

In conclusion, if we accept the premise that truth has two values and both are needed to liberate its reality, then this awareness could enhance the nursing profession, from nursing units, to board meetings, to sharing this knowledge at conventions. Think of how fruitful it would be if an orator with the values of one view would accept the fact that people with the other view cannot and will not accept the orator's argument in its raw form. Before progress can be made in oration, both will have to agree that they will disagree with each other on a raw idea and then refine it to a point of agreement.

# Chapter 22

# THE ROLE OF HEMISPHERIC PREFERENCE IN LAW PRACTICE

JAMES H. C. THOMAS, JR.

The very nature of our system of laws is to give meaning and purpose to our lives through a well defined body of law. At the same time, we are all both controlled and regulated by these laws and given the freedom and flexibility to expand our activities. By knowing the limitation of the regulations, we interact to expand our activities. In this context, the law does not set the trends in our society, but rather acts or reacts to the needs of society in regulating human conduct to meet the goals of law and order, or, in other words, meets the aims of our democratic society under our system of law.

A basic example of this regulation/interact theory is how our laws relating to the rules of the road, or operating a motor vehicle, have evolved. The numerous rules controlling speed, condition of a vehicle, driver requirements, and other restraints in operating a motor vehicle all regulate and control our driving activities to limit vehicular conduct. The benefit to society, in return, is to enlarge our freedom to use the roadways at a fairly rapid speed knowing that those around us are doing predictable things such as staying on the proper side of the road, yielding the right of way, and following the rules of the road. This gives meaning and purpose to our lives in transportation.

This same concept of meaning and purpose of law in our society may then be used in every area of our democratic civilization. Every law enacted has a purpose, limits or controls to some extent, and enlarges our interaction with others by that certain knowledge of what to expect in return. The problems that arise are due to the fact that while we are a system with laws, we are human beings in our actions. The rules of the road anticipate every possible situation where people could be injured to avoid traffic accidents, yet accidents occur every day. The explanation of accidents in traffic is that someone broke a rule of the road or was careless. This gives rise to what is called the enforceability of our laws, where one utilizes the courts to enforce a legal right against a person who has wronged them. Thus, the practice of law involves the weighing of legal rights of individuals through an adversarial proceeding as an after the fact resolution.

The Sonnier Model of Hemispheric Preference (HP, see Chap. 3), placed in this arena, reveals yet another way to examine the visual versus analytical differences in HP approaches to dealing with human problems and relationships. The very nature of legal proceedings falls well into the stereotypes of the two HP categories, both in handling of a fairly normal, or usual case, as well as in the types of cases in which attorneys choose to become involved.

Normally, a case has a complaining party, the plaintiff, confronting the offending party, the defendant. The visual HP characteristics fall comfortably into demands expected of the plaintiff's attorney of representing the cause of a person who has been wronged and seeks to have society place an interpretation on the events labeling the aggrieved conduct as a wrong and seek redress, usually in the form of monetary compensation. The case of the plaintiff is portrayed as that of one who is helpless and in need of the aid of the courts as a balancing of the rights of the parties to make whole or right a wrong.

The defendant's attorney more aptly follows the analytical HP approach by characterizing the conduct in question as very insignificant and raises the plaintiff's own misconduct as the real cause of his own injury. He may even suggest that the court leave the two parties as they found themselves and maintain a status quo in both fault and charge. To him, the procedure is a series of concerted steps to prevent or minimize any change in the status of the parties involved.

The types of cases available to the legal profession brings out the HP nature of each attorney as they choose the field in which they litigate. With the Constitution as the buttress onto which our legal system is founded, the system of laws provides a fertile ground for steady and constant change in our scheme of doing things. The traditional method of interpretation requires that one ask what the framers intended in 1787 when the document was written. This lends itself to a strictly analytical, conservative approach with little room for flexibility... it means what it says. However, the liberal interpretation, consistent with solving society's problems, holds that the Constitution is a living, viable document that serves as a guide, as intended by its framers, and is to be viewed as evolving in its interpretation as society evolves.

Obviously, the problems of a small nation in 1787, with relatively meager developed resources in its economy and people, differ vastly from the problems of the world power of today. Over the years, visually-oriented people have had a field day in applying change to the Constitution as the country evolved with all of the attendant problems presented and answered, even though there are still very basic issues pending, such as abortion, gun control, and separation of church and state.

With the development of issues such as these, and with the presence of what has been called the Third Constitution to the country, the Civil Rights Act of 1964, liberals have been able to again take on the cause of the weak and minorities to advocate and vigorously press forward with curing more social ills in ways not previously available in our scheme of laws. The analytical seethes with animosity at the inroads now available to change which were not present a short time ago. Minority rights, whether based on race, sex, economic origin, religion, or sexual preference give our already litigious society yet another arena for the human engineer to work toward a utopia of equality.

Perhaps the most obvious distinction between visual and analytical attorneys lies in how they deal with their clients. The visual attorney lays out the pros and cons of a case, the strong points and the weak, and leaves the ultimate decision to his client, who must live with the outcome. The analytical attorney takes a more direct approach and tells his client of whether the case is to be won or lost and exactly how it is to be handled, with little room for the human equation, which may ultimately play a part in its solution. The visual attorney does the work of his client with client input. The analytical attorney dictates to the client how the work is to be done. These are, of course, the two extreme values of truth. According to the Sonnier Model there are few consistent practitioners at these extremes, and most attorneys are eclectic and use both sides to the needed advantage. In most cases, the client has the counsel of his attorney and the two work together toward the client's best interest.

The bruhaha (see Chapter 1) typically provides fertile grounds for the clash of visual and analytical attorneys to meet and show their true HPs. They bring their two sides of truth as they square off and apply their respective talents and expertise in the lengthy and technical procedures leading to the final solution. Each feels that the values of his side of truth comprise the correct and proper approach. The results never deter either opponent from his feeling of righteousness. In reality, the system needs both values to balance the teetering truth of public interest because they are both a vital part of the same system.

## Chapter 23

# THE SOCIAL ASPECTS OF HEMISPHERICITY IN EDUCATION

Andrea L. Wesley

No man is an island, but each is a social being in need of others of his or her kind with whom to live and to enjoy a good quality of life. This basic need is at the very root of the challenge to educators today. The classroom is a social setting with constant verbal and nonverbal communications between teacher and pupils, as well as between the pupils themselves. If this is true, then *why* and *how* do some children, apparently bright children, fail? How can a teacher be so challenged and motivated as to meet the many different needs of all students in the classroom? Does the teacher have a personal or professional responsibility for the success or failure of all students? If so, is there a way to insure a high level of success for all teachers in reaching and teaching all students?

**Individual Differences in the Cognitive Modes of HP.** The answers to some of these questions can be based on the hemispheric preference (HP) of each teacher. For the people oriented, student centered, visual teacher, there can be no social equality in education as long as so many people doubt the fact that each teacher has a personal/professional responsibility for the success or failure of all students. For the project-oriented, subject-centered, analytical teacher, stratification is the norm. However, as wide apart as these basic viewpoints are, holistic education removes the need to focus on diversity, for its practitioners look relatively the same in their delivery modes (Sonnier, 1982b, 1985, 1989). But, until this ideal is reached, education will continue to be a hit-and-miss, affective social adventure. This reality is well expressed in the social interaction components of the two cognitive modes, visual and analytical, and is revealed in both teaching and learning styles.

**HP and the Learning Styles.** The school is indeed a social setting in which the child must constantly respond to a number of social stimuli. Among these are the inputs of the teacher, other students, and even the student himself/herself. Academic, social, and other aspects of student performance are the student's net response to all of these stimuli. Whether each teacher can give an informed and caring answer to each question depends largely on whether or not he/she realizes fully that the classroom is a social setting. With this realization comes the understanding that the student is prey to some psychological (nature) and environmental (nurture) forces which influence the communication basis of both teaching and learning styles in the social setting of the classroom.

The visual learner has difficulty in learning with abstractions and symbolisms, but does well with task-oriented learning environments. The analytical learner has the best of the situation with a setting that typically responds to his/her need for structure, order, and verbally detailed instruction. Holistic education reaches and teaches both because it is responsive to the visual hemisphere, which handles emotional, visuospatial tasks, and to the analytical hemisphere, which handles best linear-logical, verbal tasks of the traditional classroom (Sonnier, 1982b, 1985, 1989).

**HP and Teaching Styles.** Educators have long suspected that individual differences in student performance may be biologically based on differences in the manner in which information is processed. The two HP modes appear to be syncretic with two different, observable strategies for processing the information of each hemisphere. The dichotomy of constructive, analytical, verbal qualities of the left hemisphere versus the opposing creative, holistic, and visuospatial qualities of the right hemisphere are labels which appear to represent these two modes or natures of hemispheric functions (Bogen, 1977; Sonnier and Goldsmith, 1985; Sonnier, 1989).

Learning and teaching styles are examples of this dichotomy as influenced by the mediation of HP. Teachers must come to grips with these individual differences in children. The traditional teaching approach continues to result in academic failure for some and success with little effort for others. Because of these differences, instructional methods must respond to the apparent condition that some children are visually oriented while others are analytically oriented (Santos Rego et al., 1989). Holistic education is the label which Sonnier (1985) has placed on this all important endeavor to involve all parts of the individual in neuroeducation (Zenhausern, 1982).

There is widespread need to explore and correct the negative impact that some teaching styles have on some learning styles in the social educational environment. Case in point, what impact do cognitive, verbally-based strategies of analytical teachers have on the affective, visuospatial strategies of visual learners? From this perspective of "both sides of the desk," the impact is devastating for these children. Sonnier (1982b, 1985, 1989) addressed these factors as justification for the implementation of holistic education. His observation was that analytical teacher prefers teacher-oriented strategies; on the other hand, visual teachers prefer student-oriented strategies.

Instructional objectives should maximize the performance of all students and thus, should be so diverse as to meet the needs of all students. *Holistic education* has that potential in that: (1) it satisfies the needs of both visual and analytical children; (2) it helps the visual child to develop analytical skills and it helps the analytical child to develop visual skills; and (3) learning needs not met result in academic failure and in lowering of self-esteem (Santos Rego et al., 1989). The Warner Brothers movie, *Stand and Deliver*, exemplifies the positive results of holistic education.

In summary, according to Sonnier (1982b, 1985, 1989), holistic education has a number of factors which have a positive influence on the social setting of the classroom. The student learns at a more personal and gratifying manner which makes for a happier learner. Student affect soars and being there is fun. Thus, holistic education has a positive impact on both cognitive achievement and affective attainment. And, probably more important, there is the potential for visual learners to practice toward skill development in the analytical mode and for analytical learners to develop skills in the use of the visual mode.

## Chapter 24

# THE ROLE OF HEMISPHERIC PREFERENCE IN SALES PREPRESENTATIVE TRAINING

John S. Sonnier

Company executives and corporate boards market their products or services widely, but with fiscal discretion. There are two distinctly different marketing strategies and it is proposed that the proponents of these strategies are influenced by values of their hemispheric preferences (HPs). Briefly, the analytical person is generally too conservative to act on impulse and the visual person is generally too impulsive.

**HP Characteristics of Executive/Board Members.** Conservative marketing of a product limits its visibility and smothers any potential for profit gain. An example of this is the executive, or board, which usually reflects a conservative, analytical HP. Executives with these values generally have the potential for analyzing and matching a product-market, but show only a faint visibility for market expansion through sales representatives (SRs) who are equipped with written and oral information and product samples. Therefore, these persons are not likely to see the need for this kind of budget expenditure.

Persons with the opposing values have a visual HP and a better perspective for matching a product-market. However, they lack the analytical mentality needed to oversee a calculated level of budget expenditure on marketing exposure as a function of the level of both real and potential profit gain. This makes them predisposed towards squandering profit.

Coming to grips with the level of sales representation needed at any particular point of a product or service history is obviously in need of both liberal-visual and conservative-analytical input. In the light of these HPs, my objective is to describe sales representation from the moment the executive or corporate board decides to make a particular product more visible for the purpose of raising the level of profit. This process starts with the *selection* of the right person for the job, then the *training* of that person, and finally an appropriate written and oral *presentation* of the product, along with a representative sample.

## Selecting the Right Person for the Job

**HP of SRs.** Although together, they represent less than 15 percent of Sonnier's Model of Hemispheric Preference (see Chap. 3), both highly visual and highly analytical persons could make good SRs, each in their own way. Sonnier and Wesley propose that slightly visual and slightly analytical persons, from birth and by nature, pick up and display a significant number of the opposite traits and values of both hemispheres during the nurturing process. If this is the case, then the result would be the expansion of their eclectic range (see Chap. 5). This should make the interview process less of a mystery, but no less difficult. There is emphasis on the product-market that the executives wish to match or augment and the person who they deem to be best suited for the job.

During the course of a product representation visit, the highly analytical SR does and says what is needed to be done and said with the precision of a machine. He is less likely to offend anyone with his conservative and proper demure. He is more patient than his visual counterpart. However, the visual person is more apt to use ingenuity to make a floundering or failing visit work. While this SR is less organized and mechanical in tact, tactics, and demure, he is more likely to detect subtle changes and personnel qualities of the office being visited so as to make the needed adjustments in order to salvage difficult situations.

In a mutually exclusive manner, the first is more product oriented, the latter more people oriented—both good at being SRs, but different in the way they conduct their office visits. The scale of success is balanced by the reality that where one is more successful, the other is less successful. The bottom line is more than likely that analytical SRs do well with analytical clients and visual SRs do well with visual clients. An altogether different SR is the eclectic person, the swinger with both analytical and visual traits and values. While this person could be said to have the best of both worlds, the flip side is that they also share in the weaknesses of both of the hemispheric propensities.

**The Role of the Executive or Board HP(s) in SR Selection.** When making their SR selection, the two sets of traits and values of HP are reflected among the executives, as well. The person that they deem to be the right person for the job will be a reflection of the executive's or board's collective or averaged HP. The analytical, product-oriented values lean heavily toward selecting someone who is knowledgeable in the product being marketed. Visual values support the selection of a people-oriented person.

Given equal qualifications, which one should be hired? My recommendation is to bias the decision, based on need. Do you need to hire a product-knowledgable person or a trainable person who is people-oriented? Advertise the job description widely and get as diverse a field of applicants as possible. However, when interviewing, ignore the temptation to select on the basis of applicant-HP, but attempt to match a task with the person who is able, ready, and willing to implement a product-market match.

**SR Training.** A major objective for training SRs is to compensate for selection weaknesses. At least two philosophies lend themselves to the training of a successful SR. These, too, are based on the executive or board HPs, and reflect the philosophy used in the selection process. If selection was biased toward a product-oriented person, then training is needed in person-to-person behavior modification. From my experience, which may reflect my own slightly analytical HP (by nature, but people-oriented by nurture), this task is more difficult than if the bias was toward the selection of people-oriented persons. The training of a visual, people-oriented person is usually less costly in the long run because this person can learn all about the product easier through cosmetic training than an analytical, product-oriented person can learn to become people-oriented. Since there are so few highly visual and highly analytical persons to begin with, chances are that most of the candidates will be eclectic, with nature-nurture switches and blends, and either one of these could serve well with minimal training in both, people-to-people behavior modification and product cognition.

**Preservice SR Training.** One curriculum area of preservice SR training that I find lacking is a predisposition to the types of offices that the SR will be visiting in the real world. An understanding of the diversity in "atmospheres" and "types" of offices, through education, as opposed to experience, will increase a new SRs comfort level in the doctor's office. I relate to my own field of representing a prescription drug company for the product and calling on the medical profession for the market. However, this technique is applicable to a large number of other product-markets.

Doctors' offices have different "atmospheres." Some of the factors that contribute to these differences include the personality of the doctor, the staff, the specialty of the practice, the size of the group and practice, the patient population, and, among others, the geographic location of the practice. These factors of atmosphere contribute to four rather consistent "types" of offices as I perceive them, from most to least accessible. These categories are: (1) accessible physician and staff, (2) accessible physician with resistant staff, (3) accessible by appointment only, and (4) inaccessible physician.

Physicians in Categories 1, 2 and in 3 tend to be supportive and people-oriented while others in 3 and most in 4 tend to be controllers and task-oriented.

The purpose of the Preservice SR Training program is to educate new SRs to better understand and identify office types so as to maximize the benefits of such a short selling time. Category 1 is the *accessible physician and staff.* Our objective in every office visit is to get more physicians to use more of our prescription drugs. While these offices are particularly enjoyable for new SRs, the time factor is essential to continued success. They give us time and say what we like to hear. But, remember that they are as friendly to SRs from other companies. It is tempting to believe that we are the favorite SR in this office and get all of the business when in fact they may tend to spread the business so as to help everyone.

Category 2 is the *accessible physician with resistant staff.* These physicians are no different than those of Category 1. However, a hostile staff may prevent his access. Often, because of a gabby boss, the staff falls behind schedule, and this makes for hectic times and/or late hours. These offices are crucial to your product. By showing the staff that you are no threat to their time factor, the chances of seeing the physician are greatly improved.

Category 3 is *accessible by appointment only.* Because more SRs are calling on physicians than ever before, some use this method to cope with the influx. Therefore, situations where the physician needs to be seen four times per quarter could present a problem. As with Category 2, the need is to deliver brief, high impact messages in between appointments; through brochures and samples left with the nurse, and to befriend the physician so as to eliminate appointments, altogether. Category 4 is *physicians who are inaccessible.* Although these offices do not, as a rule see SRs, the staff cooperation varies. Some are friendly, but fearful of the physician. Others are cold as a reflection of the physician's demands. Most physicians who do not see SRs are task-oriented controllers and these offices can be intimidating and frustrating for new SRs.

The *action steps* for Categories 2, 3, and 4 may include any or all of these:

1. Identify the role of the staff. Who decides on your access, the receptionist, the nurse, or both?
2. Know the names of each staff member.
3. Record the physician's and staff members' birthdays, interests, hobbies, and anything about their children and inquire about these during subsequent visits.
4. Fill their walls and countertops with service items and shower them with personal items.
5. Schedule luncheon and tape showings and leave copies for the physician to study.
6. If you do get to see the physician, cut through small talk and get your message in, being mindful of and grateful to the staff.

The aim of the action steps is to let the staff and physician know that you care and to set yourself apart from the competition so as to gain accessibility. The prime objective is to move all of these offices to Category 1 status.

**Brochures, Samples and Oral Presentations.** Each product *or service* to be marketed is distinctly in need of a well designed and presented brochure. This is a costly option and should therefore be done with professional advice. A determination of the quantity and quality of the samples to be given out is also costly and should likewise be done with professional advise. The verbal presentation should be learned in training sessions.

## Conclusion

The conclusion is that it costs money to make money and the level of expenditures in profit-motivated expansion is in need of input from both visual and analytical managers. Uncontested, the analytical manager keeps a chokinghold on fiscal responsibility to a stagnation point. The visual manager dreams away at product-market matches, but may not respond to fiscal responsibility. If the theme is applied that *truth has two values,* together, they profit, and divided, or alone, they could fail.

It is clear that HP permeates the entire process from product-market management, to SR selection, marketing the product, and finally, to product sales representation. The knowledge and understanding of this phenomenon will facilitate purposeful selection of the SR and a more meaningful structuring of the training program to cover his/her weaknesses. While in training, the SR comes to grips with action steps for the various office types which will likewise facilitate a smoother entry into the service of marketing a product as its SR.

## Chapter 25

## THE ROLE OF HEMISPHERIC PREFERENCE IN UNDERSTANDING FAMILY SYSTEMIC FUNCTIONING

### Mary Ann Adams

The location of Adams's contribution among the last chapters is no indication of its significance. This is one of the most important contributions to the project that produced this book. Reviewing these ideas were for me like stroking a grandchild. In 1980, Kemp and I wrote, "Teach the Left Brain and Only the Left Brain Learns, Teach the Right Brain and Both Brains Learn." Adams's message is that to intervene in therapy through logic and reasoning is to reach only the propensities of the analytical hemisphere. However, to intervene in therapy through the visual propensities is to reach the whole person, i.e., holistically; and to reach for the whole family is to effect the total system, i.e., systemic.

I.L.S.

*Systemic family therapy* is often identified as a primary mode of intervention for family dysfunction. *Family dysfunction* is defined as marital problems, parent-children problems, or any other relationship conflict that usually stems from the absence of healthy, positive communication. The systemic approach to family dysfunctions can be closely aligned with visual hemispheric preference (HP) thought processing as proposed by Sonnier. The opposite approach to this would be analytical thought processing and would more closely align with the use of individual logic and reasoning.

**Characteristics of Visual HP.** According to Sonnier, it is characteristics of the visual preference to view the world as an environment of continual growth and change that is ever evolving through historical development. Proceeding from this source of values, the systemic approach to therapy deals with past, current, and the future of human relationships and events. This approach reveals the history of the persons involved in these relationships, as well as their dreams and aspirations for the future. In this approach to understanding family relationships, there is no such thing as absolute truth. This leads from the assumption that each person views their own truths, colored by their own experiences, feelings, and emotions of the pasts, and flavored with their own anticipations for the future (Becvar and Becvar, 1982) (see Fig. 15 for the different values of visual and analytical thought processing).

**Some Visual Techniques of the Systemic Approach.** In order to understand this relational truth, and not to be blinded by what one family member may present as absolute truth, systemic therapists typically include more than one person in the interviewing process, especially in the assessment phase of therapy. If the opportunity presents itself, several generations are included in the therapy sessions. Grandparents, in-laws, and especially children can give valuable information that assists the therapist in reconstructing, evaluating, and assessing the relationship patterns. The reconstruction of this history provides a more accurate picture of the presenting problem.

Visual techniques are often employed to assist both the therapist and the client in understanding family functioning that is based on their relational truths. The family metaphor is a commonly used visual technique in systemic therapy. When questioning family members in order to determine patterns of function, the therapist often gets bits and pieces that are a result of the family members attempting to self-analyze and to dissect their problems. The use of visual techniques, such as the metaphor, provides the therapist with the clues needed to reconstruct the broader systematic picture and to reveal the interpersonal relationships that were learned from the bits and pieces of information. After seeing this systematic picture, the smaller parts of interaction begin to make sense. For example, this is a result of the use of metaphors:

> Our family is like a refrigerator. Mom and Dad are the actual unit. The kids only come to the refrigerator when they want something. Mom and Dad are usually pretty cold and if not; if they show warmth, it is seen as a weakness. Also, Mom and Dad may constantly put their energies into storing things in the freezer compartment, not living for the present but planning for the future.

Other visual techniques employed in systemic family therapy include the following topics from Sherman and Fredman (1986): Guided Imagery— The Inner Adviser, The Empty Chair in Family Therapy, Symbolism and Gift Giving, The Family Ritual, Family Choreography, Sculpting, The Use of Dreams in Family Therapy, and among others, Poetry and Song Lyrics in Couples Groups.

| FEATURES | ANALYTICAL | VISUAL |
|---|---|---|
| CHARACTERISTICS | Views the world as complete and fixed for eternity. | Views a dynamic and evolving world through historical development. |
| | The world is marked by harmony of an objective order. | The world is marked by progressive growth and change. |
| | Speaks of the world in terms of well-defined essences using abstract, universal terms. | Speaks of the world in terms of individual traits using concrete historical concepts. |
| METHOD OF OPERATION | Begins with the abstract and derives principles from universal essence. | Begins with experience and derives accumulated experience. |
| | Deals with universals of humanhood by deriving principles from the physical nature of being human. | Deals eith the historical person in historically particular circumstances |
| | Conforms to authority and to pre-established norms. | Formulations of norms are historically conditioned |
| | Emphasis on duty and obligation to reproduce established order. | Emphasis on responsibility and actions fitting to changing times. |
| | Primarily deductive. | Primary inductive. |
| | Conclusions will remain the same. | Some conclusions will change as emperical evidence changes |
| | Conclusions are always secure as long as deductive logic is correct. | Leaving room for incompleteness, possible error, open to revision; conclusions are as accurate as evidence will allow, but these are accurate enough. |
| ADVANTAGES | Clear, simple, and sure on views of reality an conclusions about what to do. | Respects the uniquesness of the person and the peculiarities of historical circumstances |
| DISADVANTAGES | Tends to be authoritarian in the sense of claimimg to have answers suitable for all times. | Tends to be relative in the sense that everything is conditioned. |
| | Tends to be dogmatic in the sense of having the last word. | Tends to be antinomian in the sense that all laws are relative. |

## THE UNIVERSAL VIEWS RESULTING FROM VISUAL AND ANALYICAL THOUGHT PROCESSING

*Figure 15.* Visual and analytical HPs can be clearly delineated as the basis for the chemistry of group dynamics. The two different hemispheres generate mutually exclusive, universal views that in turn reflect their respective values input. For example, analytical people tend to express values from a conservative view while visual people tend to express liberally-oriented values. However, evidence is that to intervene in therapy through the visual propensities is to reach for the whole person, i.e., holistically. To reach for the whole family is to affect the whole system, i.e., systemic (adapted from Gula, 1989, pp. 32–33).

The systemic approach emphasizes the need for individuals to evolve and to take responsibility and actions to fit the changing times. Systemic therapy, therefore, is based on a family developmental framework, which establishes expectations or tasks, that lead toward the solving of normative crises. Crises can strike even when a well-functioning family moves along the aging continuum (Carter & McGoldrick, 1989). These could include crisis of the birth of the first child, the launching of the first child, children in adolescence who are breaking away, and among others, the empty nest crisis.

The well-functioning family can overcome any number of crises if they realize that crisis and coping through adaptations is a normal part of life. However, a common cause for dysfunction in families is to get "stuck" in a particular aging continuum stage and fail to adapt to the future demands. One example of these presenting problems could be the parents that still parent a sixteen-year-old as a ten-year-old child, refusing to let him/her grow up. Therefore, for families to be healthy, they must acquire a visual perspective and see life as it presents itself, continually caring and evolving. This will better enable them to adapt to the changing family life cycle.

**The Role of HP in the Systemic Approach.** Families are made up of individuals that span the spectrum of HPs from highly visual to slightly visual and from slightly analytical to highly analytical (see Chap. 3 for a discussion of this distribution). The fact that the systemic approach to family therapy reaches, involves, and heals such a wide range of human beings towards wellness is in itself an indication that the gamut of HPs are reached by the approach.

According to Sonnier and Kemp (1980), teach the left brain and only the left brain learns. But, if one teaches the right brain, both brains learn. According to this analogy, to lend intervention therapy to the analytical propensities of logic and reason would reach only analytical propensities. However, to lend intervention therapy to the visual propensities is to reach both propensities. Elsewhere, Sonnier (1982b) applied the term *holistic* to any process that simultaneously reaches both hemispheres. Reference is to the *whole person.* By this definition, the approach is holistic. This may serve as yet another view that points to the role of HP in the systemic approach to family therapy.

It is widely accepted that feelings and emotions are seated in the visual hemisphere. This, too, may help explain and lend credence to both the utility and intervening nature of visual activities in the healing process for dysfunctional families. Even though the two characteristics of visual and analytical thought processing are different, through systemic family therapy, the assumption is that both achieve their goals as family members reach a new level of communication. As individuals find understanding within themselves and among themselves, the systemic approach can create the return of a functional family.

In conclusion, my proposal is that to intervene in therapy through individual logic and reasoning is to reach only the propensities of the analytical hemisphere. However, to intervene in therapy through the visual propensities is to reach the whole person, i.e., holistically; and to reach for the whole family is to affect the total system, i.e., systemically. Family intervention therapists are invited to investigate the role of HP on family systemic functioning, as herein proposed, as well as its role in the intervention for dysfunctional families.

# Chapter 26

# AN HISTORICAL PERSPECTIVE OF HEMISPHERIC PREFERENCE IN COUNSELING

JOSEPH W. WESLEY AND ISADORE L. SONNIER

It is proposed that various personality theories and counseling applications have evolved under the influence of hemispheric preference (HP) as the driving force of their theorists/therapists. Some of the theories have evolved from a clinical setting, while others have evolved from the laboratory environment. In either case, when exploring the nature of man, some theories were guided by an analytical, rational HP of the theorists in their questions and answers about human nature. Others were forged from the same questions and answers, but influenced by the visual HP of their theorists.

Most of these theories emphasize a developmental approach to acquiring a personality, holding that human beings go through different stages as certain skills and cognitive processes are developed. However, problems emerge from insufficient mastering of one or more of these developmental stages. A common assumption is that flaws in the adult personality can be traced to aberrant internal or external, personal or environmental causes, and that individuals can be assisted, through counseling, to determine what went wrong or why they are not able to cope with their present day problems.

It is safe to say that both the questions of how each man's unique way of dealing with himself and the world about him, *theories of personality development,* and those answers that emerge as solutions to correct what has gone wrong in that development, *counseling/therapy,* reflect contrasting vantage points of the nature of man. The birth and growth of the field of psychology can be seen as a gradual progression from dealing more subjectively, as with the feelings, emotions, and other propensities of the visual hemisphere, to more objectively measurable and rational propensities, associated with the analytical hemisphere.

It is proposed that HP differences are expressed in these different philosophical concepts and the therapeutic techniques of their proponents. Placing these differences in this context may shed light both to how and why they are different. The support of this view comes from the model that therapeutic techniques can be placed on a continuum with one end being authoritarian, representing the analytical HP, while the other is nonauthoritarian, representing the visual HP on the other end, in accordance with the Sonnier Model of Hemispheric Preference (see Chap. 3). While few individuals represent one or the other of these two extreme ends, the assumption is made that these ends represent mutually exclusive forces tugging at either end on the theorists/therapists within the profession. This assumption leaves the vast majority of people as eclectic individuals on one side or the other of the continuum as determined by their dominant and nondominant HP.

In this model, a few individuals are entrenched in one or the other HP mode, often leading to misunderstanding, disbelief, disgust, and distrust of persons who have the other view. According to Sonnier and Asher (Chap. 6), the analytical hemisphere's propensities are to analyze and evaluate everything. It is sensitive to flaws, is skeptical, resists new and untried experiences, defends only familiar and ordinary circumstances, argues for the precedent to prevail, and is defensive. The visual hemisphere's propensities are to be nonevaluative or nonjudgmental, to be open, to be trusting, to show faith in the system, and to exhibit creativity.

Given the premise that a clinician has a visual HP, this propensity would leave him/her with a tendency to be more "people" oriented. The visual clinician is prompted to lead clients towards wellness by allowing them, like a bird, to fly freely in pursuit of personal goals that may be totally different from anyone else's goals and achievements. The clinician with an analytical HP, on the other hand, is more "system"-oriented, armed with a host of norms and patterned expectations. Therapeutic actions are taken in order to bring the client back into the "fold of humanity." The resulting conclusion is that the HP of the therapist determines the theory and therapy strategy which greets the client. Thus, in parallel context, it would appear that psychologists, to whom the world turns for the definition of intelligence and a definitive statement on personality development, are themselves fitted for life with one of these two modes as their dominant HP.

A widespread and influential variable in the expression of the HP of the theorist/therapist has been the behaviorist-cognitive dichotomy most highly celebrated in theories of learning and motivation. This dichotomy best parallels the continuum of opposing HPs. It is presented as a background for the counseling process as a paradoxical historical and contemporary translation of theory into practice. Although many of the therapy approaches do not indicate HP as a central premise, with the research on hemispheric dominance, we can hypothesize that those theories that emphasize verbal, learning, and highly structured environments could be classified as left hemispheric/analytical dominant. Theories that emphasize nonverbal behavior, intuition, projection, and humanistic feelings could be classified as right hemispheric/visual dominant. For example, one line of thought emerged from a group of researchers like Watson and Skinner that have come to be called behaviorists. A rather incompatible line of thought emerged from Freud and his psychoanalytic approach. Still other approaches borrow from both ends of the continuum.

Watson and Skinner emphasize mastering the environment and controlling the response to it. Images can easily be made of rigid structuring of the external world, leading to little input from the person himself. Watson and Skinner displayed examples of highly analytical theoretical tendencies. Watson expanded the classical conditioning approach to behavior change, using pain to motivate rats as well as humans to exhibit change. People may be likewise adversely influenced in preconceived therapy strategies of wellness. Skinner learned that he could more effectively bring about behavior change with manipulation through rewards rather than of punishment. His belief in social engineering and preconceived outcomes in behavior modification leaves little or no doubt about his having an analytical HP. Because of the more assertive and directed approach to counseling founded on their theories and the direction and emphasis of their thinking about personality development, it is not difficult to see why they were referred to as "behaviorists."

The heavy influence of analytical HP on this movement assured its criticism from Maslow, Rogers, and others with an apparent visual HP who are more people-oriented in a laissez faire manner. Thus, counselors of the "behavior persuasion" are often not so much concerned about why the ego develops, or why the maladapted development stages occur, as they are about what the problem is, how it was learned, and how it can be unlearned or replaced. The general emphasis that has evolved in counseling theory is to teach or somehow cause the client to undergo a behavior change.

In the historical context, the role of Freud may be viewed as a bridging of the analytical-visual continuum. His medical training and actual therapy experiences, both as client and as therapist, forged what could be viewed as a union of the behaviorist-cognitive continuum. Internal conflicts shaped the personality structure of the individual. External forces contributed as well to the adjustments to be made by this often silent, unconscious motivator guiding man's behavior.

In consideration of HP, the wide range of help received by clients through the psychoanalytic approach is suggested to be an indication that this approach moves both visual and analytical clients towards wellness. The historical perspective of Freud's HP could be viewed as slightly analytical because of his suspected vista and reach to both extremes of the continuum. A contemporary therapist, Ellis, later criticized Freud's philosophy and techniques.

Although trained in psychoanalysis, Ellis' frustration with the psychoanalytic strategy led him to study learning theories as the basis for personality development and psychotherapy. Ellis did not see any need to sit through several therapy sessions while he had already gained insight into the client's problems. From his study of learning theory, Ellis developed in 1955 his Rational Emotive Therapy approach. This approach is based on the philosophy that man is a rational being and that irrational thoughts are the cause of maladapted behavior. According to Ellis, irrational thoughts are learned and with the proper rehabilitative techniques, they can be unlearned. Ellis' techniques rely heavily on verbal processing, but involves both hemispheres. The therapist uses verbal confrontation, verbal teaching, and verbal self-talk to help the client towards behavior modification. His quicker approach to wellness differed primarily in homework assignments between therapeutic sessions.

According to Patterson (1973), Ellis indicated evidence of an analytical HP because of his approach to wellness through reason. However, his belief was that it was the client's responsibility to change from illogical to logical thinking represents conflicting evidence towards a visual HP. Thus, in accordance with the HP criteria stated above (see Chap. 3), Freud and Ellis showed indications of being slightly analytical and rather eclectic.

On the other extreme is the visual hemisphere view. These theorists emphasize the nonverbal behavior, intuition, projection, and humanistic feelings. Maslow and Rogers represent therapists with this approach. Rogers' approach can be classified as humanistic because of his belief that the individual is capable of solving his/her own problems if given the right therapeutic environment. Client independence is a major goal. Compared to Ellis, this goal is not so much a movement from the illogical to the logical, but as it is an opportunity to provided an environment for change from self-doubt and low self-esteem toward self-actualization and personal goal achievement. The main avenue for expressing these concepts is through using feeling words that the client can understand, addressing the problem that the client is presenting, and nonverbally communicating acceptance by the counselor. From this perspective, one can see that the emotions and sensory perception are a function of both hemispheres.

The conclusion is that HP may well have been a major driving force that created individual differences among counselors/therapists in the past, and so, too, with clients. It was also intended to present a possibility that different clients need different approaches toward wellness. If so, it raises many questions. What approach(es) span the range of HPs to reach most people? The idea is so novel that further investigation will be necessary to make this determination. Many other questions are raised by the HP model and await further investigation.

# BIBLIOGRAPHY

Asher, J.J. (1972). "Children's first language as a model for second language learning," *Modern Language Journal.* 56:133-139.

———. (1987). *Learning another language through actions: the complete teacher's guide* (Third Edition). Los Gatos, CA: Sky Oaks Productions, Inc.

———. (1988). *Brainswitching: a skill for the 21st century.* Los Gatos, CA: Sky Oaks Production, Inc.

Becvar, R. & Becvar, D.S. (1982). *Systems therapy and family therapy: a primer.* New York: University Press of America.

Bogen, J.E., DeZure, R., TenHouten, W.D., & Marsh, J.F. (1972). "The other side of the brain, IV: the A/P ratio," *Bulletin of the Los Angeles Neurological Society.* 37:46-61.

Bogen, J.E. (1975). "Educational aspects of hemispheric specialization," *UCLA Educator.* 17:24-32.

———. (1977). "Some educational implications of hemispheric specialization." In Wittrock, M.C. (Ed.). *The human brain* (pp. 133-153). Englewood Cliffs, NJ: Prentice-Hall.

Bosnick, A. (Ed.). (1990). "Doers of the word," *The Word Among Us.* 9:4-9.

Carter, B. & McGoldrick, M. (1989). *The changing family life cycle: a framework for family therapy.* Needham Heights, MA: Allyn and Bacon.

Cogan, M.L. (1973). *Clinical supervision.* Boston, MA: Houghton Mifflin.

Dunn, R., Cavanaugh, D.P., Eberle, B.M., & Zenhausern, R. (1977). "Hemisperic preference: the newest element of learning styles," *Journal of the National Association of Biology Teachers.* 44:291-294.

Edwards, B. (1979). *Drawing on the right side of the brain.* Los Angeles, CA: J.P. Tarcher.

Gardner, H. (1978). "What we know (and don't know) about the two halves of the brain," *Harvard Magazine.* 44:24-27.

Gazzaniga, M.S. (1975). "Review of the split brain," *UCLA Educator.* 17:9-12.

Glickman, C.D. (1990). *Supervision of instruction: A developmental approach* (2nd Ed.). Boston, MA: Allyn and Bacon.

Gula, R.M. (1989). *Reason informed by faith.* Mahwah, NY: Paulist Press.

Halberstam, D. (1969). *The best and brightest.* New York: Random House.

Harper, T.S. (1990). *Cognitive achievement with affective results in mathematics education.* Unpublished doctoral dissertation, The University of Southern Mississippi, Hattiesburg, MS.

Harrington, W.E. (1961). "First year teachers and supervision," *Ohio School Journal,* 39:32–33.

Hunter, M. (1976). *Future directions for the National Institute of Education.* Paper presented for the NIE Curriculum Development Task Force. Washington, D.C.

Keefe, J.W. (Ed.). (1982). *Student learning styles and brain behavior.* Reston, VA: National Association of Secondary School Principals.

Krashen, S.D. (1975). "The left brain," *UCLA Educator.* 17:17–23.

Lashbrook, V.J. & Lashbrook, W.B. (1980). "Social styles as a basis for adult training." Presented to Central States Speech Association, Communication Therapy Division, Chicago, IL.

Levy, J.M. (1991). *Contemporary Urban Planning.* Englewood Cliffs, NJ: Prentice-Hall.

Lortie, D.C. (1975). *School teacher: A sociological study.* Chicago, IL: University of Chicago Press.

Martin, R.A. & Yoder, E.P. (1984). *Selected supervisory techniques used by principals and their implications to success of beginning teachers.* Paper presented at the Annual Meeting of The American Educational Research Association, New Orleans, LA.

Moynihan, D.P. (1981). *A life in our times.* NY: Houghton Mifflin Co. In a review of Galbraith, J.K. (1981). *The New Yorker.* August 10, p. 103.

Nebes, R.D. (1975). "Man's so-called 'minor' hemisphere," *UCLA Educator.* 17:13–16.

Paterson, C.H. (1973). *Theories of counseling and psychology.* New York: Harper & Row Publishers.

Popham, W.A. (Filmstrip-Tape) (1969). *Instructional supervision: A criterion-referenced strategy.* Los Angeles, CA: Vimset Associates.

Reich, R. (1991). "A more perfect state of the union address," *The Wall Street Journal.* January 30, p. A-10.

Santos Rego, M.A., Doval Salgado, L., Sobrado Fernandez, L.M., & Sonnier, I.L. (1987). "A strategy for empirically evaluating holistic teaching," *Reading Improvement.* 23:277–287. See also Sonnier, I.L. (Ed.). (1989). *Affective education: methods and techniques* (pp. 131–141). Englewood Cliffs, NJ: Educational Technology Publications.

Sergiovanni, T.J. (1987). "The metaphorical use of theories and models in supervision," *Journal of Curriculum and Supervision.* 2:221–323.

Sherman, R. & Fredman, N. (198). *Handbook of structured techniques in marriage and family therapy.* Quens College, NY: Brunner/Mazel.

Snow, C.P. (1961). *Science and government.* Cambridge, MA: Harvard University Press.

Sonnier, I.L. (1982a). "Debates evolving from cerebral hemispheric research," *Journal of College Science Teaching.* 12:42–43.

———. (1982b). *Holistic education: teaching of science in the affective domain.* New York: Philosophical Library Publications.

———. (1984). "Debates updated: the educational implications of cerebral hemisphericity research," *Journal of College Science Teaching.* 13:376–378.

———. (Ed.). (1985). *Methods and techniques of holistic education.* Springfield, IL: Charles C Thomas.

———. (Ed.). (1989). *Affective education: methods and techniques.* Englewood Cliffs, NJ: Educational Technology Publications.

———. (1990). "Brain's left and right hemispheres assign liberal, conservative views," *The Student Printz,* November 29.

———. (1991a). "Brain's left and right hemispheres assign liberal, conservative views," *The Student Printz,* November 29, pp. 1, 4.

———. (1991b). "Hemisphericity: a key to understanding individual differences among teachers and learners," *Journal of Instructional Psychology.* 18:17–22.

Sonnier, I.L. & Goldsmith, J. (1985). "The pedagogy of neuroeducation: achieving holistic education." In Sonnier, I.L. *Methods and techniques of holistic education* (26–30). Springfield, IL: Charles C Thomas.

Sonnier, I.L. & Kemp, J.B. (1980). "Teach the left brain and only the left brain learns, teach the right brain and both brains learn," *The Southern Journal of Educational Research.* 14:63–70.

Sonnier, I.L., Fontecchio, G., & Dow, M.G. (1989). "Quantity and quality education: measuring affective learning." In Sonnier, I.L. *Affective education: methods and techniques* (pp. 125–130). Englewood Cliffs, NJ: Educational Technology Publications.

Sonnier, I.L., Wesselmann, D.M., & Goldsmith, J. (1985). "Introduction and overview." In Sonnier, I.L. *Methods and techniques of holistic education* (pp. 3–10). Springfield, IL: Charles C Thomas.

Spirduso, W.W. (1978). "Hemispheric lateralization and orientation in compensatory and voluntary movement." In Stelmach, G.E. (Ed). *Information processing in motor control and learning* (pp. 289–309). New York: Academic Press.

Taber, G.D. (1989). "Affective education and a nation at risk." In Sonnier, I.L. *Affective education: methods and techniques* (pp. 125–130). Englewood Cliffs, NJ: Educational Technology Publications.

Tisher, R.P. (1979). *Teacher induction: An aspect of the education and professional development of teachers.* Paper presented at the National Conference: Exploring issues in teacher education: Questions for the future, Austin, TX.

Torrence, E.P., Reynolds, C.R., Riegel, T., & Ball, O. (1977). "Your learning and thinking, Form A and B: preliminary norms, abbreviated technical notes, scoring keys, and selected references," *The Gifted Child Quarterly.* 21:563–569.

Vitale, B.M. (1982). *Unicorns are real: a right-brained approach to learning.* Rolling Hills Estate, CA: Jalmar Press.

Will, G.F. (1983). *Statecraft as soulcraft: what government does.* NY: Simon & Schuster.

Williams, H.S., Leonard, R.L., & Rose, M.D. (1990). *Role congruency between elementary school teachers and their principals: An exploratory investigation.* Paper presented at the annual meeting of The Southern Regional Council on Educational Administration, Atlanta, GA.

Williams, L.V. (1983). *Teaching for the two-sided mind: a guide to right brain/left brain education.* New York: Simon & Schuster, Inc.

Witelson, S. (1977). "Developmental dyslexia: two right hemispheres and none left," *Science.* 195:309–311.

Wittrock, M.C. (Ed.). (1977). *The human brain.* Englewood Cliffs, NJ: Prentice-Hall.

Zenhausern, R. (1982). "Education and the left hemisphere." In Keefe, J.W. (Ed.). *Student learning styles and brain behavior* (pp. 192–195). Reston, VA: National Association of Secondary School Principals.

# INDEX

## A

Adams, M.A., v, xviii, 108
Administrators/Administration, instructional, 40
 athletic, 75–77
 democratic, 60
  amenable to change, 77
  communicative, 77
  flexible, 77
  loose organization, 77
  patient, 77
  supportive, 77
  teacher-relationships, 85–87
  willing to try something different, 77
Affective attainment, 30–35, 36, 39
 positive/neutral/negative, 32
Ambidextrous, 19
Analytic/Analytical preference (see Hemisphericity/Hemispheric preference)
Arizona State University, 76
Art & science, blending, 83
Asher, J.J., v, xvii, 25, 114
Authoritarian leadership, 12
 autocratic/task-oriented, 75–76

## B

Behaviorists, 115
Bible, 67
Biology, 11
Bogen, J.E., 6, 7, 36, 100
Bosnick, A., 67, 68, 69
Boston Harbor, 28
Bowden, B., 77
Bowdoin College, 79
Brains/left-right, xiii
Bruhaha, 3, 4, 97

Bush, G., 28
Business/Firm, product/service, 63–66
 customers, 64
 decision-making, 66
 entrepreneur, 64, 65, 66
 management, internal/external, 63, 67
 needs/environment, 64
 rise and fall of, 63–66
Brain/Behavior, 37

## C

Carnagie Foundation, 42
Carter, B., 111
Cerebral hemispheres (see Hemisphericity/Hemispheric preference)
Chamberlain, J.L., 79–80
Chicago Bears, 76
Christian behavior, 66–71
 moral theology, 67–71
 personal/interpersonal, 66
Civil Rights Act of 1964, 97
Clinical Supervision Model, 42, 43
Coaches, 75–77
Cogan, M.L., 42
Cognitive/Academic achievement, 30–35, 36, 39, 44
Cognitive styles, 36
Confederate-Union, 79–80
Conflict/confrontation, ix, 18, 19, 26
Conservative input/views (see also Hemisphericity/Hemispheric preference, analytical, conservative), ix, x, 3–5, 25–27, 29, 49, 60, 61
 documents, 13, 110
 vs. the L-Word, 28–29
Constitution, 96, 97
Corpus callosum, 7
Counseling (see also Psychology), 113–117

Creativity/Creative thinking, *19*–21, 49, 53, 55, 58, 68
Criterion-Referenced Supervision, 42, 43
CSM (*see* Clinical Supervision Model)
C-RS (*see* Criterion-Referenced Supervision)

**D**

Defendant-plaintiff, 96
Democratic administration (*see* Administrators/Administration)
Developmental Supervision Theory, Glickman's, 47
Democratic leadership/Forum, 12, 27
    Egalitarian, 77
    Civilization, law in, 95
Dialogue, allowed/disallowed, ix, x
Ditka, M., 76
Domain, psychomotor, 37
Domestic policy, *61*
Dow, M.G., 40
Dunn, R.,
Dysfunction, family, *108*, 109, 111
    well-functioning, 111
Dyslexia/Dyslexics, 7, 53–54

**E**

Economy/Economics, 60–63
Education/Educational:
    affective attainment, *30*–35
    cognitive achievement, *30*–35
    dichotomy, 36
    elitist system, 49
    goals/ends, x
    holistic, *30*–35, 36, 39–47
    knowledge/understanding, ix
    implementation/management (*see* Sonnier Model of Educational Management, The)
    marketing, 66
    model (*see* Sonnier Model of Educational Management, The)
    military training, 78
    neuroeducation, 37
    photojournalism, 82
    policy/thought/practice, ix, x
    public, 85–89
    skill acquisition, 23
    social aspects of, *99*–101
    success, 25
    system, 36
    testing, standardized, 48–51
    United States, in the, 38
Edwards, B., 37
Egalitarian rule, 12, 27
    relationship-motivated, 75–77
Elementary schools/teachers, 9, 37, 38, 53
Elitist rule/system, 12, 27, 49
Ellis, H., 116, 117
Engineer, 11

**F**

Family:
    dysfunction, 108, 109, 111
    functional, 112
    systemic functioning, 108–112
    systemic therapy, 108–112
    well-functioning, 111
    whole, 112
Florida State University, 77
Fredman, N., 109
Freud, S., 116
Frey, W.W., v, xvii, 52
Fontecchio, G., 40
Foreign policy, *60*

**G**

Gardner, H., 6
Gazzaniga, M.S., 6, 7
Gettysburg, Battle of, 74
Glickman, C.D., 44, 45
    Developmental Supervision Model, 47
GNP, 61
Goldsmith, J., 39, 46, 100
Government, conservative/liberal, 69
    equity-efficiency, 61
Green Bay Packers, 76
Gula, R.M., 12, 13, 69, 70, 110

**H**

Halberstram, D., 60
Harper, T.S., 40
Harris, S., xiii
Harrington, W.E., 41

# Index

Haspeslagh, J.A., v, xviii, 91
Hemisphericity/Hemispheric preference:
   activities, ix
   achievement-oriented, 76
   analytical, ix, 6–8, 9–13, *18*–24, 25, *26, 27,*
      37–38, 43, 48–49, 58, 63, 70, 75, *78,*
      81, 82, 84, 86, 87, 96, 101, 102, 103,
      104, *110,* 113–117
      advantages, 12, *13, 110*
      attorneys, 97
      Auditory, 7–8, 11
      authoritarian, 27, 38, *75*–77
      auditory, 7–8, 11
      characteristics of, 12, *13, 110*
      Classicist Worldview, 69, *70*
      conservative, 25–29, 60, 68
      deductive, 13, 110
      dictatorship, 27
      disadvantages, 12, *13, 110*
      examine all sides, 63
      formal, 76
      highly disruptive/obstinate, reclusive, 11
      law-and-order-oriented, 72–74
      method of operation, 12, *13, 110*
      propensities, x
      risk averse, 63
      subject-centered, 31, 99
      totalitarian, 27
      wait-and-see, 63
   antagonistic value systems, ix, x, 68
   art, in Christian, 68–69
   athletic administration, in, *75*–77
   auditory, ix, 7–8, *11*
   autocratic/task-oriented, *75*–76
   awareness, 9, 42
   business management, in *63*–66
   cerebral, ix
   cognition, constructive/creative, 11, 49, 51
   cognitive mode, individual differences in, *99*
   cognitive styles, two, 36
   communicate/communicative/
      communication, x, ix, 18, 24, 25, 27,
      30, 36, 54–55, 63, 77, 99, 108
   conflict/confrontation/struggle, ix, x, 18,
      19, 26, 51, 87, 91, 93–94
   confrontation (*see* conflict/confrontation/
      struggle)
   conservative (*see* analytical, conservative)
   constructive-creative, 11, 49
   crime/criminal, *72*–74
   counseling, historical perspective of, *113*–117
   counseling/therapy, 113
   creative-constructive, 11
   criticism, 115
   curriculum preparation, in, 39
   data/findings (*see* research/findings)
   debate/disagreement, acceptable point of
      departure, 68, 74
   decision, moral, 68
   decision-making process, 66
   determination of, 9
   dichotomy, 6, 12, *36*–37, 114
   differences (*see* Hemisphericity/
      Hemispheric preference, truth, two
      sides of)
   different values (*see* Hemisphericity/
      Hemispheric preference, truth, two
      sides of)
   discovery of, *6*–7
   discrimination based on, 51
   diversity, 67
   dominant/dominance, 9, *10,* 20, 37, 63, 114
      nondominant, 9, *10,* 20, 114
      mixed, 9, 12
   eclectic blend, 37, 75, 103
   education, in public, *85*–89
      social aspects of, *99*–101
   elitist system, 12, 27, 29, 49
   engineering sciences, in, 52–55
   executive/board, role of, in, *103*–104
      characteristics of, *102*–103
   family systemic functioning, in, *108*–112
   forces, diverging/dividing (*see also* Truth,
      Two values/sides of), 68
      separately, inadequate, 68
   individual differences in (*see also* Individual differences), ix, xv
   iconoclast-iconophyle debate, 68–69
   implementation, ix, 30–35, *37*–38
   information processing, visual/analytical,
      23, 26

Hemisphericity/Hemispheric preference
    (*continued*)
  intelligence, types of, 36
  investigation of (*see* Research)
  issues, moral:
    abortion, 69
    clerical celibacy, 69
    extraordinary means to extend life, 69
    infant mortality, rate of, 61
    sexuality, 69
  knowing, ways of, 36
  lateralization, 37
  liberal (*see* Visual)
  law practice, in, *95*–*97*
  learners, 6–8, 9–13, *11*, 37, 101
  lesson planning, in, 39
  life-styles, *10*, 27, 99
  major-minor, 6
  methods and techniques of, xi
  military leadership, in, *78*–*81*
  minds, both, 49, 66
  misconceptions, ix, 6–8
  misnomer, ix, *10*–11
  misunderstanding, 18
  model (*see* Sonnier Model of Hemispheric
    Preference, The)
  moral theology, in, *67*–*71*
    Catholic, Magisterium, 67, 68, 69
    Christian/Christendom/Christianity,
      67–71
    Protestant, Bible, 67
  mutually exclusive, 12, 103
  nature/nurture, x, *8,* 10, 11, 12, 18, 20, 24,
    29, 38
    two basic natures of, 63
    nondominant, 9, *10,* 37, 63
  nondominant, 9, *10,* 20, 114
  nursing, in, *91*–*94*
  obstacles to understanding of, 6–8, 9–13
  orchestrated modes, 38
  personality development, x, 8, 12, 25
  phenomenon, ix, x, xi, 6–8, *7,* 9–13, 17, 25,
    29, 39, 48, 51, 68
  photojournalism, in, *82*–*84*
  physiological basis for, 7
  policy due to:
    polarized/failure, 60
    public formulation of, *59*–*62*
  problem solving process of, 49

product-market/service, in, 63–66
  matching, 102
propensities:
  analytical/visual, x, 14, 18, 25
  mutually exclusive, 12, 18, 103
relationship, positive:
  player-player, 77
  coach-player, 77
remediate: confrontation/strife, ix, x
research/findings, 7–8, 9, 10, 11, 14–17, 24,
  37, 40
role of, ix–xii, 12
  in sales representative training, *102*–*107,*
    103
scientists, among, *56*–*58*
selected life-styles, xix, 10, 20
self-diagnosed, 9, 10, 11
SMHP (*see* Sonnier Model of Hemispheric
  Preference, The)
social styles, 14–17
split-brain research, 7
stress, coping with, *93*–*94*
stress factor in nursing, on, *91*–*94*
struggle (*see* Conflict/confrontation/
  struggle)
students/learners, 6–8, 9–13, *11,* 37,
  39
supervisors, 45
task-motivated, 76
teachers/teaching, ix, *11,* 36, 38
  student-centered, 12, 37
  teacher-centered, 12, 37
  styles, 100
tenent for, 36
testing, standardized, 48–51
traits, 12, 19, 25
training of sales representatives, in, *102*–
  107, *103*
truth, two values/sides of, x, xi, xiii, xv,
  *3*–*5,* 6–8, 18, 19, 24, 29, 56, 58, 63, 66,
  67, 68, 72, 73, 78, 81, 90, 93, 96, 104,
  114, 117
understanding:
  analytical preference, *22*–*23*
  two preferences, the, *18*–*19*
  visual preference, *18*–*19*
  HP in coping with stress, *93*–*94*
unity-disunity due to, x
universal views, xix, 13, 70, 110

Hemisphericity/Hemispheric preference
(*continued*)
  utopia of equity, 97, 98
  values conflict in, amalgamated, 69
  visual, ix, 6–8, 9–13, *18–24, 26, 27,* 37–38, 44, 48–49, 58, 60, 64, 70, 77, 78, 81, 82, 84, 86, 96, 101, 102, 103, 104, *110,* 113–117
    advantages, 12, *13, 110*
    attorneys, 97
    characteristics, 12, *13, 110*
    creative, 68, 85, 86, 87
    democratic (*see* Administrators/Administration)
    disadvantages, 12, *13, 110*
    highly disruptive/obstinate/reclusive, 11
    humanistic (*see* Humanistic tendencies)
    inductive, 113, 110
    informal, 76
    laissez faire, 115
    liberal/the L-Word, *25–27,* 61–68
    method of operation, 12, *13, 110*
    Modern Worldviews, 69, *70*
    nonreaders, 7
    open/trusting, 68, 77
    people-oriented, 31, 99, 115
    previsualization photography, 82, 84
    rehabilitation-oriented, 72–74
    student-centered, 31, 38
    tendencies (*see* Humanistic tendencies)
  works, contrasting, 25
Hewlett Packard, 66
Holistic educator/education, ix, xi, xii, 24, 30–35, *36,* 38, 40, 55, 57
  affective attainment, 30–35, 40–47, 101
  cognitive achievement, 30–35, 40–47, 101
  implementation, 38, *44,* 89
  mandated: visual aids/thorough explanation, 43
  philosophy, 39–40
  positive aspects/impact/influence, 101
  skill development, 101
  supervision of, instructional, *39–47, 43*
  removes HP differences, 43–44, 92, 101
  research/findings, 40
  test for HP in, ix–x, xi–xii

Whole mind/Whole person/whole child, x, 36, *39,* 40
Holtz, L., 77
Horton, W., 28
HP (*see* Hemisphericity/Hemispheric preference)
HUD/S&L scandals, 29
Humanistic perspective, tendencies, 61
  agreeable, 77
  considerate, 77
  friendly, 77
  harmonious, 77
  paternalistic, 77
  pleasant, 77
  relaxed, 77
  sincere, 77
  warm, 77
Humanitarianism, 29
Hunter, M., 39

**I**

IBM, 66
Indiana University, 76
Individual differences, ix, xi, 6–8, 19, *25–27,* 29, 30, 38, 39
  hemispheric preference, the basis for, 30
Innovation (*see* Creativity/Creative thinking)
Intellectual talents/skills, 51
Institutional management, ix, x, 68, 73
  forces vital to, xi, xv
Institution/society, ix, xi, 6
  administration, 77
  democratic, ix, x
  economics, ix
  educational, ix, x, xi, 73
  human, ix
  improvement, 41
  management, ix, xv
  political, 6
  social, ix, xi
Instructional supervision (*see also* Sonnier Model of Educational Management, The), 12, *39–47, 41, 42, 43*
  characteristics, 39–47
  Developmental:
    interpersonal skills, directive/collaborative/nondirective, 45

Instructional supervision (*continued*)
  holistic education, for, *43*–44
  model (*see also* Sonnier Model of Educational Management, The), 40, 41
    dominant model, 42
    strategies, 47
    student-centered, 42
    teacher-centered, 42
    mismatch, 42
Instructional techniques:
  traditional/holistic, 40
  windows/walls, 43

## J

Jordan, Michael, 83

## K

Keefe, J.W., 6
Kemp, J.B., 46, 108, 111
Kennedy, J.F., 24
Knight, B., 76
Krashen, S.D., 6
Kush, F., 76

## L

L-word, the (*see* libral views/input)
Larkin, G.R., v, xviii, 59
Larkin, M.J., v, xviii, 85
LaSorta, T., 77
Lashbrook, V.J., 14
Lashbrook, W.B., 14
Law, regulation/interact theory, in, 95
Law enforcement, 72, 73, 74
Leadership, conservative/analytical, 55
Learning outcomes (*see* Sonnier Model of Educational Management, The)
Learning styles/strategies:
  auditory/analytical, ix, 6–8, 9–13, 37, 49, 101
  environment, 32
  hemispheric preference among, *11*
  individual differences in, 39
  process, 36
  students', 37, 39
  systems, 37
  visual, ix, 6–8, 9–13, 37, 38, 50, 101

Lecture, 32
Leonard, R.L., 41
Levy, J.M., 61
Lewis, C.W., 18, 24
Libral views/input (*see also* Hemisphericity/Hemispheric preference, visual liberal), ix, x, *3*–5, 12, *25-27*, *29*, 60, 61
  L–Word, the, *25*–*29*
  documents, 13, 110
  humanitarian, 27
  visual, 55
Life Magazine, 83
Life-styles, *10*, 20
Litigious society, minority rights arena:
  race/sex/economic origin/religion/sexual preference, 97
  human engineer, 97
  utopia of equity, 97
Lombardi, V., 76
Lortie, D.C., 41
Los Angeles Dodgers, 77

## M

Management:
  business, 63–66
  educational, *30*–*37*
  institutional, 51, 68, 73
  mismanagement, 74
Marketing strategies, 102
Martin, B., 76
Martin, R.A., 41, 42
Maslow, A., 115, 116
McElroy, M., vi, xvii, 18
McGoldrick, M.,
McNamara, R., 60
Medicine/Medical, 24
Military leadership/history, *78*–81
Monologue, ix, x
Movie, *Stand and Deliver*, 6, 30, 44, 50
Moynihan, D.P., 59

## N

National Commission on Excellence in Education, 42
National Institute of Education, 39
Nationalism, 27
Nebes, R.D., 6, 7

# Index

New York Yankees, 76, 77
Nobel Prize, 36
Notre Dame, 77
Nurse-patient relations, *92*
Nurse-supervisor relations, *92-93*

## P

Panko, T.R., vi, xviii, 72
Paterno, J., 77
Patterson, C.H., 116
Patton, G.S., 80-81
Penal code, 73
Pennsylvania State University, 77
Photojournalism, *82*, 84
Physicians, 103, 105, 106
Plaintiff-defendant, 96
Personality development, x, 8, 12, 25
    maladapted, 115
    theories of, 113-114
Politics/Political, ix, 6, 24
    conservative/liberal, 25-29
Policy:
    public/political/failed, 60
    foreign, *60*
    domestic, *61*
    rational/analytical/successful, 60
Poole, W.H., III, vi, xvii, 75
Popham, W.A., 42
Principal-teacher transactions, 46-47
Protestant, 67
Psychology, birth/growth of, 113-117
    counseling, *113-117*
Psychomotor domain, 37
Punishment, 72, 73

## R

Reading, *21*
Reality (*see* Hemisphericity/Hemispheric preference, truth, two sides of)
Regulation/interact theory in law, 95
Rehabilitation, 72-74
Reich, R., 61
Research (*see* Hemisphericity/Hemispheric preference, research/findings)
Republican administration, 60
Rogers, C., 115, 116
Rose, M.D., 41

Rule:
    dictatorship/totalatarian, 27
    egalitarian, 12, 27
    elitist, 12, 27

## S

S&L/HUD scandals, 29
Sales representative training, 102-107
Sanity, mathematical, 60
Santos Rego, M.A., 33, 36, 101
Schools, elementary/secondary/undergraduate, 53
Science and art, blending of, 83
Science education/educators, 53, 58
Science/Technology, 56-58
Scientific enterprise, 58
Scientific evidence, 9
Scientific Research Society, The, xiii
Self-actualization, 10
Self-esteem/respect, x, 10, 72
    low, 10
Sergiovanni, T.J., 41, 42, 43
Sherman, R., 109
Sigma Xi, xiii
Skinner, B.F., 115
SMEM (*see* Sonnier Model of Educational Management)
SMHP (*see* Sonnier Model of Hemispheric Preference)
Smith, E., 83
Smith, W.C., vi, xviii, 63
Snow, C.P., 59
Social aspects in education, *99-101*
Social confrontation/order-disorder, 26, 29, 72
Social scientists, 60
Social styles, 14-17, *21*, 23
    analytical/amiable/driver/expressive, 16
    assertiveness/responsiveness, 16
Social styles profile, 14
    specialists: supportive/control/social/technical, 15
Society, litigous, 97
Sonnier, C.B., vi, xvii, 30
Sonnier, D.L., vi, xviii, 78
Sonnier, I.L., vi, xvii, xviii, 3, 6-8, 9-13, 14, 18, 25, 30, 36, 39, 40, *41-47*, 49, 54, 55, 56, 57, 59, 62, 63, 72, 90, 92, 99, 100, 101, 103, 108, 111, 113, 114

Sonnier, J.S., vi, xviii, 102
Sonnier Model of Educational Management (SMEM), The, xvii, 30–35, 43–44, 45, 46, 47, 55
   *Category 1* of the, 31–35, *33*, 40, 41, 42, 44
   data collection forms, *34–35*, 42
   Design/treatment, 33–34
   Four Categories of, 30–*31*, *41*
   implementing the, *44*–47
   Instructional supervision, *39*–47, *41*, 42, *43*
   maintenance of, *35*
   rationale, *31*–32
   student checklist, *32*
Sonnier Model of Hemispheric Preference (SMHP), The, xi, xvii, 9–13, 14, 25, 56, 58, 91, 96, 101, 103, 114
Southerland, A.R., vi, xvii, 48
Spirduso, W.W., 37
Sperry, R., 36
Split-brain research, 7
*Stand and Deliver*, Warner Brothers Movie, 8, 30, 44, 50, 101.
Steinbrenner, G., 76
Stengal, C., 77
Struggle (*see* Hemisphericity/Hemispheric preference, conflict)
Student learning/enjoying, 30–35, 39–47
Student, observations of, *37*
Supervision, instructional (*see* Instructional supervision)
Systemic approach, visual technique in family therapy, *108, 109*, 111, 112

## T

Taber, G.D., 42
Teacher: preservice/inservice, 9, 40
   administrator relations, *85*–87
   elementary, 9, 37, 38
   effectiveness, 30–35, 36, 39–47
   holistic techniques/strategies, 43
   observations of, *37*
   professional development, 44
   student/pupil transactions/relationships, 46–47, 88, *91*–92
   teacher relationships, *87*–88
   special education, 88–89

Teaching method/Strategy, x, xii, 30–35, 41
   analytical/authoritarian, 38
   environment, 32
   hemispheric preference in, 11
   process, 36
   supervision, 39–47
   traditional, 30–35
   visual/self-directed, 38
Testing, standardized, 48–51
   built-in bias, 48, 49
      discriminates against visuals, 48
      racial/cultural, 51
   negative outcomes, 48
Tests, lengthy, 49
Thomas, Charles C, Publisher, xi
Thomas, J.H.C., Jr., vi, xviii, 95
Three-M, 66
Timeframe, *19*–20
Tisher, R.P., 41
Torrence, E.P., 37
Traditional teaching, 30–35, 40
   America, in, 61
   antagonistic, 60
   democratizing, 60
Truth, two values/sides of (*see* Hemisphericity/Hemispheric preference, truth)

## U

UCLA Educator, 36
Union-Confederate, 79–80

## V

Values of truth (*see* Hemisphericity/Hemispheric preference, truth)
Vietnam, 60
Visionaries, 50
Vision, 65
Visual/Libral, 29, 61
Visual aids/materials and teaching aids, 32, 36, 43, 46
Visual preference (*see* Hemisphericity/Hemispheric preference)
Vitale, B.M., 7, 37

## W

Watson, J.B., 115
Wesley, A.L., vii, xvii, xviii, 14, 99
Wesley, J.W., vii, xviii, 113
Wesselman, D.M., 39
Wheeler, E.L., vii, xviii, 82
Will, G.F., 59
Williams, H.S., vii, xvii, 39, 41
Williams, L.V., 7, 37

Wilson Learning Corporation, 14
Witelson, S., 7, 21
Wittrock, M.C., 36

## Y

Yoder, E.P., 41, 42

## Z

Zenhausern, R., 37, 100